Colostrum: Man's First Food The White Gold Discovery

by

Bernard Jensen, Ph.D.

PUBLISHED BY:

Bernard Jensen, Ph.D.
24360 Old Wagon Road
Escondido, CA 92027 USA

The medical and health procedures in this book are based on the training, personal experience and research of the author. Because each person and situation is unique, the publisher urges the reader to check with a qualified health professional before using any procedure where there is any question as to its appropriateness. The publisher does not advocate the use of any particular diet or supplement, but believes the information presented in this book should be available to the public.

Because there is always some risk involved, the author/publisher is not responsible for any adverse effects or consequences from the use of any of the suggestions or procedures in this book. Please do not use the book if you are unwilling to assume the risk. Feel free to consult a physician or other qualified health professional. It is a sign of wisdom—not cowardice—to seek a second or third opinion.

Published by Bernard Jensen
24360 Old Wagon Road
Escondido, CA 92027 USA

ISBN 0-932615-28-70

WHAT'S IN THIS BOOK

This is a book full of fascinating surprises about a healing food you are going to thoroughly enjoy reading about. This is a food so familiar to most of us, yet so little understood until recent times, that it is almost stunning to find out about its extraordinary healing influence on the body. Over 2,000 research papers published over the past 20 years verify its known properties and hint at good things yet to come.

Reports that colostrum helps rheumatoid arthritis, multiple sclerosis, candida albicans, diabetes and destroys many kinds of viruses and bacteria are presented. The protection of the bowel wall from harmful bacteria like E. coli and its toxic wastes is described. The presence of an insulin-like factor in colostrum that speeds up healing of damaged tissue is verified. The way colostrum strengthens the human immune system is described.

When Dr. Jensen announces, "There's a new star on the health food horizon," health-wise people must sit up and take notice. This book should be required reading for everyone interested in wellness and the reversal of disease. As Dr. Jensen would say, "Where there's a problem, there's a solution right beside it," and this new food could be the solution to the health problems of millions. With the U.S. people at an all-time risk for an all-time high number of deadly diseases and maladies at outrageously high health care costs, a simple, natural remedy shows promise of being one of the most effective health-enhancing and protecting foods of all time.

ACKNOWLEDGMENT

I would like to acknowledge contributions by Kim Matteo and Drs. Robert Plymate and Robert Preston, whose assistance in the completion of this book were invaluable.

DEDICATION

I dedicate this book to all the mothers who have that 100% love for their children to give them all that is needed for healthy bodies and lives.

CONTENTS

Introduction

Recently, I've made one of the most exciting food discoveries of my life, but before I tell you about it, I want to share one of the secrets of my success as a clinical nutritionist.

Throughout my over 50 years in the healing art, I have searched the world over for the best foods to build and sustain a healthy life, and my search has been fruitful, as thousands of my patients and hundreds of thousands of readers of my books on nutrition can testify. I have found many valuable, health-building foods from places like the Orient, Mideast and Latin America, as well as my own back yard.

In recent years, my lifetime of seeking and discovering foods and other aids to health and healing has begun to bear fruit of another kind: the dawning of a certain wisdom, the uncovering of principles that shed light not only on what foods heal but why foods heal and why we need healing foods so desperately in our time.

If you grasp the real-life impact of this wisdom, you will see how your life is personally involved, and you will begin to have a very different outlook on what you eat from day to day. To help get my idea across, I want to introduce you to "kingdom thinking."

KINGDOM THINKING

A kingdom, by the simple virtue of its meaning, is a domain where a king rules. The king's power has great influence over everything in his kingdom, influencing the welfare of his people, the state of their satisfaction in life, their education, health, prosperity and a host of other factors. Everything a king does is important because it has such a far-reaching effect on his domain. A king needs a healthy body, healthy mind and healthy spirit to maintain an orderly, healthy, prosperous kingdom.

The Creator has made each of us king or queen over our domain of responsibility, which includes what we add to or take from the health of the planet on which we live.

No king or queen can be healthy or accomplish anything significant unless he is energized by the proper fuel, and for man, that fuel is the food we eat. Low-energy food produces low-energy people, people without the power to prosper, avoid disease or even survive. Mankind is facing a challenge to its survival. With the whole world facing massive food shortages due to erosion losses and mineral depletion of its topsoil, food quality and availability are diminishing fast. Nations that have plenty to eat—like ours—show evidence of malnutrition by the shocking abundance of diseases related to overeating nutrient-poor food. Third World countries face problems like drought, poverty, starvation and the diseases that go with them.

The real tragedy is that you can't have a healthy mind in an unhealthy body and you can't have a healthy body with deficient and chemically-polluted foods, polluted air and polluted water. What have we gotten ourselves into?

We seem to have entered an era of planetary twilight where everything that can go wrong is going wrong. You probably know people whose lives have become disrupted by drugs, out-of-control sex, serious disease, social neglect and self-destructive lifestyles. Perhaps there are members of your own family who need help. What can we do to save ourselves and our planet? Where can we stop and take our stand for a way out of this planetary (but also very personal) nightmare?

We need to start by upgrading our own health, our own nutrition, our own strength. Man is made from the "dust of the earth," as the Good Book says, but we don't feed ourselves directly from the mineral kingdom but from the food kingdoms of this planet. When people eat right, they think right, feel right and begin to act right. They have healthier relationships. They make sounder decisions, plan with greater foresight, work with greater motivation and skill.

Healthy people say "no" to drugs, "no" to destructive lifestyle habits and "no" to trashing our beautiful planet. Healthy people have the power to take dominion over their planet and change the future. To begin this process, we need to understand and use the best, most nutritionally worthwhile foods available—foods that will detoxify our bodies, make up for long-standing nutritional deficiencies, reverse disease processes and build strong, clean new tissue in place of the old.

PLANETARY FOOD QUALITY

Before man so badly depleted and poisoned his lovely planet, we could have used many more of the foods of this earth. But, now so many foods are almost nutritionally worthless that we need to be very choosy about what we buy and eat. We need to eat more of the top foods in each kingdom, the best and most reliable foods.

We find that the Creator is concerned about the health and well-being of mankind, because He created everything we would need to prosper and be in good health. Man, himself, was created so his physical body would be nourished and protected from disease by those foods that the Creator made for him, but not by foods that would harm his body. For example, a tree-ripened apricot is approved by this standard. A pickled beet is not. A baked potato is approved, but a bag of potato chips cooked in boiling grease and saturated with salt is not. Our basic food law is that all our foods should be whole, pure and natural. That's the way it was in the Garden of Eden. Even if we can't keep this rule exactly, we should stay as close to it as we can.

Unless man eats right and follows other health laws, his exercise of dominion over the planet will fail and he will become as extinct as the dinosaurs that once lumbered so innocently over the face of this earth. *What are the best foods?* The best foods can be determined by a principle so simple that most nutritionists have overlooked it. The best foods are the foods that help us retain youthfulness and the power that goes with youth. These foods are, themselves, foods at the peak of their nutritional value. *They are foods closely related to the reproductive cycle of their kind.*

I'm talking about foods like raw seeds, eggs, whole grains, codfish roe, royal jelly, bee pollen, sprouts, fresh goat milk and edible algae like chlorella. Each of these foods is closely related to the reproductive cycle of its kingdom.

However, of all the foods I know, colostrum, which is what this book is about, has the greatest spectrum of health-protecting and health-enhancing benefits. And I have written this little book to tell you why I'm excited about colostrum, the first food of man.

Doctors and "modern" mothers argued that breast feeding was inconvenient, nutritionally unreliable and too time consuming, thus bringing about the "bottle revolution" of the 1940s and 1950s. Milk substitute manufacturers claimed their products were better—nutritionally superior to mother's milk and more easily digested.

The facts, however, finally emerged over the years as studies were done comparing nursing mothers with non-nursing mothers and breast-fed babies with bottle-fed babies. Let's have a quick glimpse at some of the things they found out.

THE ADVANTAGES TO THE MOTHER

Breast feeding benefits the mother in several ways. First, the suckling of the newborn infant stimulates the release of a hormone from the hypothalamus of the brain which, in turn, stimulates the shrinking of the mother's uterus (enlarged during childbirth), back to normal.

Second, the act of breast feeding is commonly reported to lead to a satisfying sense of peace and well-being on the part of the mother. Nursing usually develops a close emotional bonding between mother and child.

Perhaps because human mothers, like all mammalian mothers, were created and designed to breast feed their offspring, we may be missing other simple, but important, psychological benefits to the mother. Are mothers who nurse happier mothers? It would be interesting to know.

THE ADVANTAGES TO THE BABY

Not only does human mothers' milk provide the baby with the right kind of digestible proteins, but breast-fed babies are less likely to become overweight than bottle-fed babies. Studies have shown that bottle-fed babies tend to get fatter and stay fatter than breast-fed babies. There is a tendency in mothers feeding their babies by bottle to encourage them to drink it all, even though the infant may be satisfied with half or two-thirds of the bottle.

Nursing mothers can't really tell how much milk their baby has taken, so when the baby is done, so is mom. But, the non-nursing mother often jiggles her baby to wake up or to start sucking again, and croons and coaxes the babe until the bottle is dry. This programs the baby to eat past the "full" feeling, to eat more than it wants or needs.

Breast-fed babies have fewer colds, less colic and croup than bottle-fed babies. They are, on the average, stronger and healthier than bottle-fed babies, not just in the early months of life, but later on as well.

When breast-fed babies get to be school age, they are faster learners than bottle-fed babies. They are psychologically more stable, form friendships more easily and adjust to change more rapidly.

Doctors have long known that the "first milk" of new mothers, the milk given the first three days of nursing, was not only different from normal milk but had something to do with passing along the mother's immunity toward certain diseases to their newborn babies. More recently, researchers have made some exciting discoveries about this "first milk," and I'll let you know all about it in the next chapter. But now, let's see, in the chart on the following page, how human breast milk compares with cow's milk and goat's milk.

Notice that the protein in breast milk is almost one-third that of goat's milk and one-fourth that of cow's milk, while the total carbohydrate is significantly higher. The lactose content of mother's milk is about twice that of cow's milk. I have often pointed out to mothers and mothers-to-be that cow's milk was designed for creatures with hairy hides, big bones and hooves. (Notice how much more calcium there is in cow's milk and goat's milk than breast milk!) Other differences are also evident, even to the most casual eye!

MOTHER'S MILK IS BEST

I don't mean to upset anyone, but human milk is best for human babies. That doesn't mean I don't know lots of happy, well adjusted, intelligent adults who were bottle-fed babies. Statistics and averages always hide the exceptions. In general, I am convinced that babies do better with breast milk, especially considering the "first milk" (which isn't really milk at all) and its role of defending the newborn against potentially deadly microorganisms.

In the first chapter, you're going to find out what's so great about that special "first milk" of mothers, and how adults are going to benefit as well as children from a wonderful new healing food!

Comparison of Nutrients in Milk

ITEM All Items Per Liter		Breast Milk	Goat's Milk	Cow's Milk
Energy	Kcal	710	670	660
Protein	gm	11	32	42
Fat	gm	38	40	37
Carbohydrate	gm	68	46	49
Calcium	mg	340	1290	1430
Phosphorus	mg	140	1060	1120
Sodium	meq	7	15	27
Potassium	meq	13	46	45
Iron	mg	5	1	0.5
Zinc	mg	3.5	2.4	3.5
Chloride	mg	375-450	1200	1050
Magnesium	mg	46	100-145	120
Vitamins				
A	I.U.	2000	2074	1500
B-1	mg	0.160	0.400	0.440
B-2	mg	0.360	0.1840	0.2100
B-3 (Niacin)	mg	1.47	1.9	1.0
B-6	mg	0.100	0.70	0.640
B-12	mcg	0.3	0.6	4.3
Pantothenate	mg	1.84	3.4	3.5
Folacin	mcg	52	6	55
Diotin	mcg	8	39	31
Choline	mg	90	150	121
Inositol	mg	330	210	110
C	mg	43	15	21
D	I.U.	22	24	14*
E	I.U	1.8	—	0.4
Essential Fatty Acids, per 100 gm of Milk Fat			4.1	2.6
Percent Fat Globules Less Than 3 dram			63	43

*Not Fortified

CHAPTER 1

ARE YOU READY TO MEET A MIRACLE?

I must tell you, there is a wonderful new food star on the nutritional horizon, a healing food as old as mankind, as fresh and new as a newborn baby, more potent in more ways than any other food I know.

This food is colostrum.

Colostrum is the secretion formed in a female's (human or animal) mammary glands before her baby is born; it is a highly-nutritious food more potent than milk. It is the food every breast-fed baby will get in the first few days of its life before the mother's milk comes in. It is the most important food the newborn infant will ever get.

Why is it so important? Because it contains substances that provide temporary immunity against many diseases and afflictions until the baby's own immune system "turns on." It contains substances that destroy viruses. It also starts proper bowel movements, imparts the desirable acidophilus bacteria to the baby's bowel, stimulates physical growth and initiates many other body functions. One researcher has estimated that colostrum triggers at least fifty processes and functions in the newborn that provide lasting benefits, some lifelong.

More recently, we have found that colostrum has great health benefits for adults.

HOW I FIRST ENCOUNTERED COLOSTRUM

One of the great men who influenced my life and work was Dr. John Harvey Kellogg, who once received an urgent phone call from the Canadian doctor who delivered the famous Dionne quintuplets. Dr. Kellogg was asked to rush a quantity of lactobacillus acidophilus to Canada, as two of the quintuplets were having bowel problems. Possibly the mother didn't have enough colostrum for all five of her new baby girls. Acidophilus, like colostrum, helps the bowel work right. The two "quints," as they called them, pulled through.

Not much was known about colostrum at the time, except that it was important in getting the newborn's bowel started right. In fact, not much was known about colostrum until recent years, when a revival of interest in breast feeding triggered renewed interest and research in the advantages and disadvantages of breast feeding versus bottle feeding.

When doctors realized that breast-fed babies were healthier than bottle-fed babies, they began to look into the reasons why.

The question was, "What is it about breast feeding and mother's milk that makes these good things happen?"

A few doctors credited the physical closeness of mother and child for the benefits of breast feeding.

But, others began to wonder whether the colostrum had a part in the benefits. Now, after 40 years of research, we are just beginning to understand what a wonderful health-building food colostrum is.

YES, BUT WHAT IS COLOSTRUM?

Colostrum is a non-milk, breast secretion produced by all mammalian mothers for the first two or three days after giving birth. It is much higher in protein, lower in fat and sugar, than milk. It has 10 to 17 times the iron content of milk, 3 times as much vitamin D and 10 times more vitamin A.

The definition of colostrum as cited from ***Taber's Cyclopedic Medical Dictionary, Ed. 16***, reads: "Breast fluid that may be secreted from the second trimester of pregnancy onward, but is most particularly noted in the first 2-3 days after birth and before the onset of true lactation. This thin, yellowish fluid contains a great quantity of proteins and calories in addition to antibodies and lymphocytes."

The protein in colostrum is mostly immunoglobulins, from which antibodies are formed, which protect the newborn from disease until its own immune system is working. (Before birth, the mother's immunoglobulins and antibodies pass through the placenta to protect the fetus.) Human babies with defective immune systems have remained alive as long as two or three years, protected by the immune factors from the mother's colostrum.

Colostrum proteins also include hormones, enzymes, complex sugars and growth factor which speeds up the growth or healing of tissue. It contains proline-rich polypeptides to normalize an overactive or underactive immune system. It has peroxidase enzyme, which destroys disease-carrying microbes and lactoferrin which is able to neutralize some kinds of bacteria. Nucleotides provide the raw materials for building or repair of the nucleic material (DNA and RNA) in cells.

In other words, colostrum contributes many powerful health-building and protective factors to the newborn animal or child.

Researchers in the 1970s discovered the reason why colostrum is only secreted from the mother's breasts the first few days of the newborn's life. Immunoglobulins are made of proteins and are very large. During the first day or two, the newborn's intestinal wall has a limited number of enlarged pores which allow the large immunoglobulin molecules to pass through the bowel wall and into the bloodstream and lymph. These molecules become an immediate part of the protective immune system of the infant's body.

Because of the closing up of the bowel's enlarged pores after 24 to 36 hours, many scientists thought that colostrum would do little good, if used after that time. But a British doctor named David Tyrrell made an interesting discovery in the late 1970s.

Dr. Tyrrell found that the greatest protection provided by the immune factors of the colostrum was not in the blood or lymph systems *but inside the intestine and inside the bronchi, the hollow branches of the lungs. This means that people of any age can benefit from taking colostrum.*

BOVINE COLOSTRUM WORKS EVEN BETTER

We have found that colostrum from cows is even more potent for humans than colostrum from mother's milk, and can be taken by people of any age with excellent results. The cow colostrum is processed, dried into a powder and is now beginning to be available in health food stores. It is much higher in immune factors than human mothers' colostrum.

For example, a human mother's colostrum contains only 2% of IgG, the most important immunoglobulin in the body. Cow colostrum contains 86% IgG. Colostrum from human mothers would be very expensive and hard to obtain. Fortunately, bovine colostrum is easily available in large quantities.

Bovine colostrum can be used to promote passive immunity and interspecies immunity, because the colostrum of cows is accepted by virtually all other mammals including man. The disease-resistant factors in the colostrum are simply transferred to the person (or other animal) who uses it. The anaphylactic shock problem is bypassed because bovine colostrum contains a blocking hormone to keep the calf from being sensitized to its own mother's immune factors. So, anyone can use colostrum without risk, as far as we know.

I want to change the subject slightly to make a very important point. My own research and experience show that most abnormal processes that eventually develop into diseases start in the bowel (usually triggered by dietary deficiencies). It is very important to realize that colostrum can neutralize these disease processes. If we can cleanse or counteract the septic conditions in the bowel, we can protect the body from, perhaps, 80% or more of all serious disease processes. Because of the inherent relationship between the bowel and the lungs and bronchials, disease conditions initiated in the bowel often affect the lungs. The lungs should give us very few problems if we take care of the bowel. I highly recommend my book ***Tissue Cleansing Through Bowel Management***, which provides a thorough explanation of why we need to take care of the bowel and how that can be done.

We find that the bowel and the lungs, in fact, have their own immune systems, geared for the unique conditions in each type of tissue. The Peyer's Patches in the intestine and a similar system in the lungs constantly work to protect the tissue by responding to pathogenic organisms, toxins (often the metabolic wastes of bacteria are highly toxic) and allergens.

In recent years, the flood of antibiotics, sulfa drugs and antihistamines has virtually destroyed the beneficial bacteria in the bowel, allowing highly-toxic conditions and virulent germ life to take over. As antibiotics are used, immune function is lowered. When the antibiotics are stopped, the immune system is weak and vulnerable until it builds back up again. There is an urgent need to clean up this disease-promoting condition before a degenerative disease takes over. There is only so much toxicity and germ life the bowel can take care of before the lungs and bronchials are affected, at a time when immune function is too low to be any help.

As scientists have found out, colostrum is a most helpful substance for greatly improving the level of protection for the bowel and lungs in adults. I can tell you, the toxic overload in the average bowel today is so great that normal defenses such as Peyer's patches, and normal cleansing processes, such as the acidophilus bacteria, are at the point of being overwhelmed, if they have not already been overwhelmed.

Let's examine the ingredients of dried colostrum.

COMPOSITION OF DRY COLOSTRUM
(Obtained from Cows)

Protein	33.8%
Fat	01.4%
Nonfat solids	98.6%
Ash	11.1%
Lactose	29.0%
Immunoglobulins:	
IgG	87 mg/100 ml
IgA	51 mg/100 ml
IgM	131 mg/100 ml

No coliform bacteria or salmonella were found in this test.

HORMONES IN COLOSTRUM

Both hormones and prostaglandins have been found in colostrum. Hormones include estrone, estriol and estradiol. The names of the prostaglandins found were not given.

ARE THERE VITAMINS IN COLOSTRUM?

The main vitamins in colostrum produced from cows are vitamins A, B-12 and E. There are other vitamins in traces.

WHAT ELSE DOES COLOSTRUM HAVE IN IT?

The colostrum sold in health food stores contains several types of immunoglobulins, many nucleotides, orotic acid, enzymes and leukocytes capable of producing an interferon-like activity. Adenosine monophosphate is the most important nucleotide because it is transformed into adenosine diphosphate, which is involved in the body's energy production. Interferon is important because it slows virus multiplication by protecting the cells in which the virus attempts to multiply.

A study by Dr. J. F. Ballard in 1982 showed that cows' colostrum was 100 times more potent than human colostrum. There is also an ingredient in colostrum that is sufficiently similar to insulin in that it reduces the need for insulin in diabetics who begin to use the colostrum.

LOOKING BACK IN TIME

It may be that some of the ancient physicians like Hippocrates or Galen knew about colostrum, but it was not until the 20th century that the technology was developed to understand immunity.

By 1945, at least one researcher was discussing whether colostrum milk would be helpful in the treatment of diseases and ailments. Six years later, another researcher came up with an idea for enhancing the immune value of colostrum by inoculating a cow with a vaccine for a specific virus. This could be a way of making sure the colostrum produced by a specific cow would be effective against a specific virus. The same man had the idea of injecting a cow with certain antigens (allergy-producing agents) so the cow would develop the right antibodies to destroy these antigens. Then when a person began to react to the same antigens, he could use some colostrum from that cow, knowing that the antibodies would take care of the problem. These speculations have turned out to be true, as we will see later.

Now, when health care costs are higher than at any other time in history, and health problems are epidemic in proportion, a broad-spectrum health builder like colostrum offers a great blessing to mankind.

Let's take a closer look at colostrum, which we can now see has great promise as a health-enhancing and immunity-boosting food for all ages of people.

CHAPTER 2

WHITE GOLD?

When a new health product appears on the market, I always wonder, as you probably do, whether the stuff is any good or not. New products are often accompanied by advertising that exaggerates the benefits to be expected, so you don't really know whether to believe it or not.

What I like to know is, who else believes in this product? Who believes in colostrum?

If I find out that reputable people have been involved in the research, testing and production of a new product, I really get interested!

A recent magazine article titled "White Gold?" tells us that biotech companies are currently evaluating cow colostrum to see if it can be substituted for cow serum as a medium to grow mammalian cells in research or production laboratories. Cow serum from fetal calves costs about $60-$100 a half liter and is still going up. But in the 1970s, a Harvard Medical School research scientist, Dr. Michael Klagsbrun, found that mammalian cells grew especially well in colostrum, which contains a higher level of growth factor than in blood serum. Dr. Klagsbrun patented his growth medium, and at least one biotech firm has purchased a license to use Dr. Klagbrun's medium.

The magazine article confirms that colostrum is high in growth factor, which speeds up tissue repair in tissues damaged by ulcers, cysts, lesions, trauma or disease. It doesn't discuss what would happen if I took cow colostrum supplements, but it does let me know that the growth factor in it really works.

But, here's another article from an Australian newspaper that really got me interested and excited. Here's the headline and part of the article.

Adelaide Team's Growth Drug Passes Trials

A potentially life-saving drug developed by Adelaide scientists to speed recovery from surgery, accidents and existing diseases has passed preclinical trials.

Three of the scientists will fly to the United States this month to discuss the next multimillion dollar development stage with the Genentech Corporation of San Francisco.

The scientists are Dr. John Ballard, assistant chief of the CSIRO's Adelaide-based human nutrition division; Dr. Leanna Read, director of the Child Health Research Institute in Adelaide; and, Dr. John Wallace, reader in biochemistry at the University of Adelaide.

Together with Dr. Julian Wells, also a reader in biochemistry at the University, they have used genetic engineering to produce a potent, insulin-like growth factor.

Dr. Ballard and Dr. Wallace first identified the factor five years ago in the colostrum of cattle. Colostrum is the first liquid produced by female mammals in the first few days after birth and before the main milk flow.

Growth factors work mainly on muscles and connective tissue, speeding healing and halting or even reversing muscle wastage. They can also be used to cut costs in the biotechnology industry by speeding the growth of cells in tissue cultures.

Isn't that something? They started with the growth-factor in cow colostrum, then changed it through genetic engineering, possibly to make it more potent than the natural product or else to reduce the cost of producing the substance. Now they are hoping to complete their research and estimate eventual sales at $250 million per year. But, I want to tell you, I would rather use the natural product any day than use a drug made to do the same thing.

WE'D BETTER STOP, LOOK AND LISTEN

I believe drugs are useful for life-saving emergencies or when other more natural methods have been exhausted, but there are serious problems with drugs—all drugs.

Drugs have side effects, long-term effects and time-bomb effects. They are capable of combining with previously existing drug residues, heavy metals, chemical food additives and other substances in the bowel or in the body tissues to produce an extremely toxic effect or carcinogen. Drugs always do some damage to the body and should be avoided except as a last resort.

When the natural product is available, I will always use it in preference over a drug product. It is also worth considering that when you take out one ingredient from colostrum, which comes naturally with many ingredients, any symbiotic effects are removed. Often, biologically active ingredients in foods work together in harmony to produce a more profound healing or restoring effect than the same ingredients would show if used separately. Sometimes a single ingredient, taken from its usual companions, will have undesirable side effects that aren't present when the whole food is taken.

THE ANTI-VIRAL ACTIVITY IN COLOSTRUM

I have to say that I don't know how to discuss the natural anti-viral activity in colostrum accurately without appearing to praise it too much. Colostrum is loaded with immunoglobulins, from which antibodies are formed, and antibodies are especially adapted to destroy viruses.

Viruses are the most dangerous threat to world health today, and colostrum is one of the few substances that can stop them from progressing in the body. Colds, flu, herpes and AIDS are caused by viruses, and there is no known cure for any of them yet. Dr. Isaac Asimov, author of hundreds of science and science fiction books, had this to say some years ago at The World Congress on the Virus in San Diego: "It is still possible for viruses to kill millions, tens of millions, maybe hundreds of millions every year." Viruses mutate, so it is almost impossible to develop a drug that can also control the new forms a virus may take.

Antibiotics, the so-called miracle drugs used to combat so many bacterial illnesses, can't harm a single known virus. Most virus-caused diseases can only be treated for their symptoms. How does our body's natural immune system kill them? We find that antibodies made from immunoglobulins can destroy them. I want to point out that only antibodies, tailor-made to match any virus, can keep up with the viruses' tendency to mutate.

The prestigious Center for Disease Control in Atlanta, Georgia, asked Dr. E.L. Palmer to prepare a report for them on colostrum. In his report, handed to the CDC in 1980, Dr. Palmer said, "It is now well-known that a wide range of anti-viral factors are present in colostrum." We will look into the ways antibodies deal with viruses later on. It is important, however, to notice that colostrum is recognized by reputable doctors and scientists as a true health-building food.

CAN ANYTHING MATCH SULFUR?

Antibodies are made from immunoglobulins, composed of protein. The protein is made of amino acids, of which the cystine, methionine and glutathionine contain some sulfur. Dr. Kenneth Brockman believes the primary active component of antibodies, beside globulins, is sulfur, a mineral very important to metabolism. He says, "The sulfur content in colostrum enhances the natural antibiotic immune response in the body."

We'll be discussing the fascinating story of the antibody-antigen conflict later.

REPAIR AND REPLACEMENT OF DNA AND RNA

Dr. Benjamin Frank, whose research on youth and aging showed RNA to be one of the most important youth-preserving factors in human nutrition, encouraged his patients to eat more RNA-rich foods to maintain wellness, keep up their energy levels and stay younger longer. He found sardines and other fish and seafood to be very high in RNA. I have found the edible alga chlorella to be even higher. Colostrum may be even more effective in building health than chlorella.

Colostrum contains growth factors that apparently stimulate growth and repair of key nucleic materials such as DNA and RNA. Researchers have found that protein destruction is inhibited and protein repair is stimulated by an insulin-like growth factor from colostrum. The stimulation of repair includes stimulation of DNA synthesis, with RNA synthesis implied.

I feel the future may show that colostrum promotes youthfulness and retards aging. Some scientists say that many aging processes are promoted as our natural immune system is depleted. We find out that this process of depletion is reversed as colostrum has its broad-spectrum effect in building up, not only the immune system, but every organ, gland and tissue in the body that helps support the natural defenses.

For many years, I have taught that longevity and quality of life are enhanced, not by taking care of disease symptoms, but by taking care of the whole person on the other end of those symptoms. This is the true path to longevity, which is simply another word for prolonged youthfulness.

A WONDERFUL TESTIMONY

One of the most wonderful testimonies I have encountered is that of Dr. Robert Preston from Northern California, whose experience with people who have taken colostrum is most enlightening.

A 72-year-old man, wheelchair-bound with rheumatoid arthritis, began taking one tablet of dried colostrum twice a day. A week later, he came to Dr. Preston's office very excited. "I'm free of pain and I can walk," he said. Many practitioners in the healing arts say rheumatoid arthritis can't be helped, because it involves an immune system attack against the body tissue, especially in the joints. If colostrum can help reverse rheumatoid arthritis in a crippled 72-year-old, and have him up and walking in a week, it must have the ability to normalize an out-of-balance immune system.

In another case, a woman with multiple sclerosis had declined to the stage where she was confined to a wheelchair. Multiple sclerosis is the name given to the condition in which the myelin sheath that protects the nerves, and through which the nerves are fed, is gradually destroyed. When this sheath is eaten away, the nerve inside can't work properly. This causes terrible pain as it destroys muscle coordination and prevents various specialized organ tissues from doing their jobs. Multiple sclerosis often attacks nerve sheaths here and there in the body, resulting in a patchwork of muscle groups that no longer work because the exposed nerves are no longer able to conduct nerve messages.

After two weeks, this woman with multiple sclerosis called Dr. Preston on the telephone to tell him something was happening. The pain was diminishing. In four weeks, she had improved enough to get out of her wheelchair. Soon after that, she was able to take a shower by herself, for the first time in years!

Like rheumatoid arthritis, multiple sclerosis is considered an autoimmune disease, a disease caused by the immune system going out of control and attacking some part of the body. There are other auto-immune diseases which include the following:

Allergies. Immune system overreacts to an antigen.

Pernicious anemia. Immune system destroys some components necessary to make red blood cells.

Diabetes mellitus, type 1. Cells that make insulin are destroyed.

Graves' disease. Receptors for thyroid-stimulating hormones and anti-thyroid-stimulating hormones are destroyed by antibodies, resulting in goiter.

Lupus erythematosis. Antibodies destroy DNA and cell nucleii, which, in turn, destroys the organs and tissues of which the cells are made up.

Myasthenia gravis. Receptor cells for the neurotransmitter chemical acetylcholine are wiped out.

It is possible that a proline-rich polypeptide, discovered in colostrum independently by researchers in Poland and at the University of Alabama, will be helpful in reversing or alleviating these autoimmune diseases. This is most likely the substance in the colostrum that helped the man crippled by rheumatoid arthritis and the woman who had multiple sclerosis. Research has shown that this proline-rich substance helps to normalize the immune system whether it is overactive or underactive.

The two types of growth factor in colostrum should also help repair the damage of auto-immune diseases. In lupus, for example, skin cells are sometimes destroyed, a condition which the epithelial growth factor should help reverse. Epithelial growth factor may also prevent scarring of the skin in cases of severe burns or accidents. Transforming growth factor, found in two forms in colostrum, is expected to help reverse protein breakdown and stimulate repair, as I have mentioned before, in almost any part of the body.

Dr. Preston has encouraged many in the healing arts to look into the beneficial properties of colostrum.

THE SPARK-PLUG EFFECT

Dr. Robert Plymate became interested in colostrum as a consequence of his Norwegian grandparents using it as a healing food. He was aware of its potential importance as he studied animal husbandry at Reich College in Mason City, Iowa, and later conducted numerous "home" experiments, until he was convinced that colostrum needed closer study by professional researchers to prove its worth to mankind.

His home experiments and preliminary studies gave him the ammunition needed to promote more complex colostrum research projects in colleges and universities with the scientists and laboratory facilities needed to prove the healing properties of this unusual food.

Dr. Plymate was successful in promoting colostrum research at John F. Kennedy College, the University of Arizona, the University of Nebraska at Lincoln, the University of Manitoba at Winnepeg and the State University of New York (SUNY).

He has been a great spark plug in stimulating interest and research in colostrum.

Are you beginning to see why I consider colostrum a wonderful new star on the nutrition horizon? There are other reasons as well, which we'll discuss soon.

CHAPTER 3

THE TRUTH AND NOTHING BUT THE TRUTH

The colostrum from cows has been carefully studied as a result of interest in its health applications. In our previous chapters, I have described the contents of colostrum in some detail. In this chapter, I will review the scientific evidence that colostrum both protects from disease and assists in the reversal of disease, and I will explain exactly what antibodies are and what they do when a dangerous virus enters the body.

Dry cow colostrum is about 33% protein, of which over 50% is made up of immunoglobulins. I am going to explain these immunoglobulins, but I first want to make sure you understand how I view so-called disease processes.

OUR BASIC VULNERABILITY TO DISEASE

Every human being is born with a combination of genetically-inherited constitutional strengths and weaknesses. To put it very simply, it is the constitutional strengths that uphold health in the body, and it is the constitutional weaknesses that allow a disease to develop when conditions are "ripe."

In their book, ***The Truth About AIDS***, Ann Giudici Feltner and William A. Check wrote, "It has been said that each of us is born with the disease that will cause our deaths. What this means is that the genetic pattern inherited from our parents is unique to each individual. Coded on it are our biological strengths and weaknesses...." However, our secondary source of vulnerability after genetic inheritance is our lifestyle—how we choose to eat, what we choose to do with our bodies and take into our bodies, where we decide to live, how much stress we are willing to take on ourselves. We can take good care of our inherent weaknesses or we can choose to neglect or abuse them, to our own ultimate harm.

The two primary conditions that allow a disease to develop in our bodies are nutritional deficiencies and toxic accumulations in the tissues. The nutritional deficiencies always damage the constitutionally weak organs, glands and tissues the most, and when the structure and function of the constitutionally weak tissue become depressed due to localized starvation, toxic wastes accumulate in the weakened tissue, adding to the destruction and inviting disease.

Researchers have found that nutritional deficiencies impair and depress immune function while they impair and depress inherently weak tissues. As I understand it, the immune system would normally rid the body of toxic wastes that accumulate in deficiency-damaged tissues, but it can't do the job if its own activity is limited due to chemical deficiencies. So, toxic materials accumulate in the constitutionally weak tissues, not just metabolic wastes but such things as drug residues, heavy metals, cigarette smoke chemical residues, chemicals from food additives, pollutants from air and water and so forth.

When tissue becomes damaged and infused with toxic accumulations, the scavengers of nature come along to feed on the dead and dying debris. These are the bacteria and viruses. If some sort of intervention is not made at this point to reverse the situation, a person could be well on his way to a disease.

The onset and progressive development of most, if not all, degenerative diseases is either preceded or accompanied by a lowering of immune system function. Our bodies are designed to recognize and resist or destroy the so-called disease producing agents. Only the suppression of our immune system can explain why this doesn't happen.

A friend of mine has said that the suppression of the human immune system is the greatest single cause of degenerative disease in our time. We suppress our immune systems by overwork, unhappiness, stress, poor diet, excessive exposure to pollutants, lack of exercise and health-destroying lifestyle habits. There is a solution to this kind of thing. Stop doing those things that are dragging you down. Learn how to get healthy and stay healthy, then practice what you've learned. Make this your new lifestyle.

In my research, I have verified Dr. William Albrecht's teaching, "Disease preys on an undernourished body." As a clinical nutritionist, I have often been able to reverse the course of a disease by teaching my patients the value of a balanced food regimen, regular exercise, adequate rest, fresh air, relaxation and recreation. Foods are a key to the process of reversing or preventing disease.

TWO VULNERABLE SYSTEMS

Over the years, I have found two body systems to be more underactive and therefore more vulnerable to disease than any others. One is the gastrointestinal system, the most chronically abused system in the average human body, and the other is the respiratory system, which becomes underactive due to the "overflow" of waste from the gastrointestinal system. Yet, powerful immune defenses are also at work in these two systems.

In my view, then, the process of disease requires:
1) genetically inherited, constitutionally weak tissue;
2) nutritional deficiencies due to inadequate diet; 3) toxic accumulations due to tissue underactivity; 4) suppression of the immune system; and 5) a causal agent such as a metabolic abnormality, virus, fungus or bacteria. The actual disease

developmental process is somewhat more complex than this, but this is the basic framework.

GENERAL DEFENSES OF THE BODY

The disease-producing organisms people are exposed to, which I have called "the scavengers of nature," are technically called pathogens, but sometimes the highly-toxic metabolic waste products of these microorganisms cause problems too. Whatever the cause, our body defenses against disease can be divided into two types: general and specific. There are three main general lines of defense of the body: physical, chemical and antimicrobial. All of them work together to prevent disease.

Physical Defenses. The skin is a two-layered, tough, outer membrane that acts as a barrier to bacteria, viruses, parasites and many other microorganisms. When the skin is broken, pathogens such as staphylococci may enter the break and start an infection. Damp skin also attracts various types of fungus, especially in warm climates.

Mucous membranes that line the nasal and respiratory passages, the digestive system and colon, the urinary tract and other orifices that connect the inside of the body with the outside are double-layered like the skin, but not as reliable at keeping germs out. The reason is that the interior orifices or passages are warm and coated with a liquid mucus which keeps them from getting dry. Many pathogens thrive in these warm, moist conditions. When enough of them gather, they sometimes break through the membrane. Injury or irritation, sometimes due to microorganism toxic waste products, allow breakthroughs by microorganisms. Viruses can tunnel through the mucous membranes, in many cases.

Tears contain a chemical (lysozyme) that is capable of destroying some bacteria. Often, however, tears wash away any irritating substances or bacteria that gather on the surface of the eyeball.

Saliva traps and expels pathogens and helps keep the mouth from becoming a breeding ground for them.

Mucus-coated nasal hairs trap germs, pollutants and small particles from the air we breathe and pollutants.

Cilia are hairlike projections that guard the upper respiratory tract. They help move dust and germs trapped in the mucous lining of the bronchials toward the throat, where they are either swallowed or expelled as phlegm. Coughing and sneezing help get rid of mucus-trapped pathogens.

Urinary passages are cleansed by the flow of urine, which keeps the mucous membranes of those passages free of germlife.

The bowel, known to be the most polluted part of the human body, is considered one of the primary entranceways for disease-causing pathogens and for the toxins that enter the bloodstream, depress the immune system and prepare the way for future diseases. The faster the bowel transit time, the cleaner the bowel will be—within limits, of course. The mucous lining of the bowel, while intended as a barrier to disease, is more often a breeding ground for undesirable bacteria and other unhealthy bowel flora.

Chemical Defenses. Not only the skin, but its acidity (between 3 and 5 pH) keeps many bacteria and other microorganisms from collecting there. The sebum from the skin's oil glands is made of fatty acids that destroy bacteria like those that cause strep throat and scarlet fever. Perspiration contains an enzyme called lysozyme that eats through the cell walls of bacteria. This same enzyme is found in nasal catarrh, saliva, tears and tissue fluid, and it destroys microorganisms that do not belong in the body wherever it is found.

Gastric juice, dominated chemically by a very strong hydrochloric acid (pH 1.2-3.0), is able to destroy almost all bacteria and their toxic wastes. However, it allows the friendly lactobacillus acidophilus (meaning acid-loving) to pass into the small intestines without being destroyed.

Antimicrobial Proteins. There are three well-known proteins beside the globulins, which I'll discuss later, that work in opposition to microorganisms in our immune systems.

Complement is found in blood serum. It received its name because it takes part in immune system reactions involving antibodies. It "complements" or "helps out" the antibodies in those reactions. Complement is made up of 20 different proteins, which help destroy viruses and other germ life already "stuck to antibodies," in the antibody-antigen interaction. They are also able to "call" leukocytes to assist in the process of dealing with infection.

Properdin is a protein found in blood serum that works with complement to destroy various types of bacteria by attracting special white blood cells to consume them.

Interferon has become famous because it has been used in treating the AIDS virus. It usually works well against viruses, by hindering their reproduction. It is known to slow down and reduce the power of virus infections such as AIDS, rabies, shingles, chicken pox and herpes, under favorable conditions.

INTERNAL BODY DEFENSES

When an antigen enters the body, whether it is a bacteria, virus or paint speck, it soon encounters one of our millions of defenders of the body, called leukocytes, which are white blood cells. There are many different white blood cell types in the body, but this is not the place for a detailed discussion of them. Here I will present a kind of outline summary.

White blood cells can multiply very quickly in times of acute infection. An elevated white blood cell count on a laboratory blood test indicates that infection is present. I should say here that red blood cells do not participate in the defense of the body—only white blood cells do.

There are many kinds of cells that participate in keeping the body free of invading antigens, and basically they do it by surrounding the unwanted antigen and destroying it chemically. This is called phagocytosis.

Some white cells stay in fixed locations in the lymph nodes, in lymph tissue, in the liver (Kupffer cells) or in the bowel (Peyer's Patches). These cells grab and destroy bacteria and debris as they pass by in the lymph or blood.

Other white blood cells travel throughout the lymph and blood circulatory systems, destroying antigens where they find them. Through a series of chemical signals, infection in any part of the body quickly attracts millions of mobile white blood cells, which attempt to take care of the infection.

Some bacteria are able to resist the immune defenses, until a multi-step reaction is set up to kill them. Cancer cells are known to be destroyed by specialized cells called "killer T-cells," but a recent experiment showed that the presence of cancer cells stimulated a reaction in growth hormone that mobilized large numbers of cells called "polymorphonuclear leukocytes" to come and engulf the cancer cells. Apparently, small numbers of cancer cells are constantly being destroyed in the body, and it is only when conditions are favorable that they gain a foothold in the body and multiply.

However, the white blood cells can do very little to stop a virus. This usually takes a defender called an antibody.

ANTIGEN-ANTIBODY REACTIONS

Antibodies can attach to and destroy bacteria and bacterial toxic wastes as well as viruses. Unlike white blood cells that will "grab and destroy" any foreign invading microorganism or substance, antibodies are made to find and destroy specific substances only. An antigen is any kind of bacteria, virus, allergen or foreign substance that doesn't belong in the body.

In general, a virus is a strand of DNA or RNA surrounded by a bit of protein, which can only reproduce by entering a cell and utilizing the cell's processes and protein to multiply itself. The host cell is destroyed as the virus multiplies.

Since about 16% of the dry colostrum is made up of immunoglobulins, let's discuss them and their role in immune defense. Globulins are a group of proteins soluble in dilute salt solutions but not in pure water. They make up 45% of the proteins in blood serum and include immunoglobulins, lipoproteins, transferin and fibrinogen (which form blood clots).

Five different classes of antibodies, or immunoglobulins, exist in humans. They are abbreviated "Ig," which stands for *immunoglobulin* and are distinguished from one another by an added capital letter. The five classes are known as: IgG, IgA, IgM, IgD and IgE. IgA, IgE and IgG are very large molecules with molecular weights of 150,000 or more. IgM is an enormous molecule with a molecular weight of 900,000. The molecular weight of IgD is unknown. Each has its own structure and job to do in the body. These antibodies are made of protein chains called "polypeptides," the chains being made of "links" of amino acids—hundreds of them.

The immunoglobulin most commonly found in the blood and lymph is IgG, which is effective at neutralizing toxins. One type of IgA found in saliva, tears and mucus is called Secretory IgA (S-IgA). There is a second type of IgA in the body. IgM is used to destroy bacteria. (I have put them in the order of greatest abundance in the serum.) IgD and IgE are usually low in humans. IgA and IgM both require sulfur in their structure.

Each immunoglobulin can be produced in many different types, each type able to attach to and destroy or immobilize a specific antigen. There are two types of IgA which are tagged as IgA-1 and IgA-2. This IgA is made in lymph tissue lining the bowel wall, the lungs and bronchials and the genitourinary tract. IgA combines with secretory IgA which exists in tears, saliva, mucus in the nose, bronchials and vagina, and in prostatic fluid. The mucous membranes of the body are not simply physical barriers to pathogens but are coated with IgA antibodies living in the mucus, which destroy or immobilize harmful organisms trying to get into the body. But, if pathogens get past the IgA and into the body, they have to face IgG and IgM antibodies.

Most antibodies have two places on their structure where they can bind to antigens, the germs, viruses, fungi or foreign particles that do not belong in the body. Circulating antibodies are particularly effective at destroying bacteria and viruses. This is called humeral immunity. The fungi, parasites, cellular virus infections, cancer cells and foreign substances are taken out of commission by several types of lymphocytes (white blood cells) that attach to them and destroy them. This is called cellular immunity.

Many times lymph nodes intercept dangerous substances being carried along in the lymph vessels and destroy them. I don't want to discuss the whole subject of immunity here, but I do want to give you an idea of what some of the colostrum ingredients, especially antibodies, do to protect us.

There are thousands of different B-cells in the immune system, located in lymph nodes, the spleen, Peyer's Patches in the intestines and in the lungs. When a lymphocyte captures an antigen (such as a bacteria) and "shows it" to B-cells, then some of the B-cells are activated to produce antibodies able to destroy that particular bacteria.

All undesirable microorganisms or particles of matter that enter the body are classed as antigens. Many antigens can only be destroyed by antibodies "tailor-made," so to speak, to attach to and destroy that particular antigen. In other words, an antibody in the bloodstream or lymph can't kill just any bacteria or virus, but only certain types or individuals. Antigens have to come in contact with and activate a B-cell before it can produce antibodies—immunoglobulins. A person who is over-reactive to an antigen is said to be allergic to that substance. IgE and IgG-4 are the general causes of allergy overreaction to antigens in "immediate response". Delayed response allergies, which are more typical of reactions to foods, take place when IgG-4 antibodies react with the antigen.

When a person—or cow—has been infected with influenza, diphtheria or tetanus, it may carry immunity to those diseases for months or years. In the case of chicken pox, measles and yellow fever, acquired immunity may last a lifetime. This is one kind of immunity carried by the colostrum, which contains antibodies of classes IgG, IgA and IgM.

HOW DO THE IMMUNE FACTORS IN COLOSTRUM HELP US?

One of the most common undesirable bacteria found in the bowel is E. coli. It has several varieties, some of which are very dangerous. Diarrhea, urinary tract infections and other problems are caused by E. coli. Also, its metabolic wastes are so toxic that the bowel wall is irritated wherever E. coli is found.

At the University of Alabama, ingredients of colostrum, such as IgA, lactoferrin and peroxidase, were found very effective against E. coli. Research at the University of Science and Technology in France, showed that IgG and other proteins in colostrum prevented the growth and multiplication of E. coli. Immune factors in colostrum prevented the E. coli (and its highly-toxic waste) from attaching to the bowel wall, thus preventing irritation and diarrhea.

Both IgA antibodies and IgG antibodies were demonstrated to protect against cholera through colostrum. In India, the colostrum of human mothers exposed to cholera contained antibodies that prevented adherence of cholera to the bowel wall. At Children's Hospital at Ohio State University, colostrum from cows exposed to cholera protected children against contracting cholera.

Clostridium is a family of bacteria whose members include tetanus and botulism, both of which have taken many lives. Studies at the University of Texas Medical School and in a Japanese institute by a group of researchers directed by Dr. N. Wada showed that colostrum was able to neutralize the purified or crude toxins from *Clostridium difficile*.

Streptococcal pneumonia is generally recognized as a particularly serious type of pneumonia, but Swedish researchers at the University of Goteborg found out that non-immunoglobin substances in colostrum blocked the strep bacteria from sticking to the epithelial tissue of the lungs. The same substance is said to be effective against middle ear infection.

Three doctors at the State University of New York at Buffalo—Drs. Ogra, Losonsky and Fishaut—have listed a number of bacteria that are controlled by the antibodies in colostrum. They include *E. coli, Salmonella, Shigella, V. cholera, Bacteriodes fragilis, Streptococcus pneumoniae, Bordiella pertussis, Clostridium diptheriae, Clostridium tetani* and *Streptococcus mutans*.

The evidence here is very conclusive that the immune factors in colostrum help control bacteria.

Now I want to make something very clear here. These experiments come from all over the world, and there is no way that the colostrum in different parts of the world—or even different parts of the United States—will protect against the same diseases or organisms. The reason is that the animals whose colostrum is used in the experiments are exposed to different diseases in different places, and only immune factors to those diseases to which the animals have been exposed will be in their colostrum. The same is true for the cows in the U.S. dairies. Their colostrum will not all be the same.

Another thing I want to point out. Most of the experiments claimed only that the colostrum was *bacteriostatic*, that is, capable of limiting the growth and multiplication. Two experiments claimed "bacteriocidal" and "antibiotic" properties for the colostrum.

I believe colostrum will strengthen a person's resistance against any bacterial infection, but I don't believe researchers are saying that ingredients in colostrum are sufficient to destroy all the undesirable bacteria. Perhaps this is for the best, because the body's own immune system must be exercised and strengthened by doing some of the work.

ANTI-VIRUS ACTIVITY OF COLOSTRUM

The most common virus activities in humans produce colds and flu, and the organisms that cause these change so frequently that new antibodies have to be developed in our bodies every time we get them. On the other hand, colds and flu are rare among those who keep themselves in top physical condition. But there are other viruses that occasionally try to pose as guests in the human body, and we will find that colostrum does quite well in evicting them.

In 1980, Dr. David Tyrrell of the Clinical Research Center and Worthwick Park Hospital in Harrow, England, showed that antibodies from IgA in colostrum could attach to the surface of viruses and prevent infection, but without the production of complement and other processes that usually accompany antigen-antibody reactions. Oligosaccharides and polysaccharides in colostrum also counteract viruses.

Bronchitis and pneumonia are often initiated by a virus called respiratory syncytial virus. After exposure to this virus, both humans and animals had protective antibodies against it in their colostrum. These were of the IgA and IgG classes.

Diarrhea and bowel inflammation may be the result of exposure to rotavirus. Japanese doctors who gave cows a strain of rotavirus along with their feed found powerful antibodies against this virus in their colostrum. When this colostrum was fed to people with bowel problems, it prevented their usual diarrhea and IBS (irritable bowel syndrome).

The Echo virus can cause a type of meningitis, while the Coxsackie virus causes a disease like polio but without paralysis. According to Dr. R. H. Michaels, immune factors in colostrum are able to neutralize the effects of these viruses.

After an experiment in which they tested colostrum against several known bowel viruses, Dr. E. L. Palmer and his associates agreed that "a wide range of antiviral factors are present in colostrum and milk."

In the 1950s and 1960s, Dr. Albert Sabin, who developed a polio vaccine, claimed he had found antipolio virus antibodies in cow colostrum, even though cows were not known to get polio. When used by humans, the colostrum protected them from getting polio.

Cells infected with Herpes Simplex virus were destroyed when colostral cells and antibody were used in an experiment conducted by Dr. S. Kuhl and his associates at the University of Texas Medical School at Houston, Texas.

I have no doubt that colostrum is effective against many types of viruses, as these studies show. Notice that researchers are not saying that colostrum immune factors are effective against every type of virus. But, they help a great deal on several significant diseases.

Let's finish the chapter by looking at three more useful discoveries concerning the ability of colostrum to protect from disease.

THREE FINAL EXPERIMENTS

AIDS headlines have made an obscure substance called interferon famous, because interferon was expected to lengthen the lifetime of those with the terminal AIDS disease.

Interferon is produced, under certain conditions, by lymphocytes. This chemical interferes with a virus' ability to grow and multiply, which means that it can't spread and take over lots of other cells. The secretion of interferon caused by the presence of one virus *also protects cells from other unrelated viruses in the vicinity*. Interferon doesn't kill viruses, it just prevents their spread, which is still a tremendous help.

Research at the University of Hong Kong in the late 1970s showed that colostrum contained leukocytes (white blood cells) which could make interferon just as well as blood-circulated lymphocytes, under the right conditions.

A second experiment by the same Hong Kong researchers was published in ***Pediatrics*** in 1978, showing the presence of leukocytes in colostrum that were effective in controlling the yeast infection of *Candida albicans*. Other researchers at the State University at New York claimed to have found in colostrum specific antibodies against *Candida albicans*. With all the difficulty we've seen in finding a natural cure for *Candida*, the results of these experiments are good news.

Third, an insulin-like effect has been found in colostrum. While researchers are hesitant to say that colostrum contains insulin, the activity of the substance is comparable to the insulin derived from pigs, which is marketed commercially. The strength of this "insulin-like" substance in colostrum is 100 times greater than the insulin level in the blood of the cows that produced the colostrum.

EXPERIMENTS WORTH GETTING EXCITED ABOUT

In my opinion, the preceding described experiments, all performed by highly-trained researchers, many of them at prestigious institutions, show that colostrum is the most promising health food product in many years. I am, personally, excited and enthusiastic about it, and I hope you are too.

I believe scientists will continue to tap the secrets of this ancient remedy in years to come, but we know enough about it now to see that it is effective in preventing and reversing disease.

CHAPTER 4

COLOSTRUM CASE HISTORIES

One of the pioneers of colostrum research in our time has been Dr. Robert Plymate, whose influence has stimulated many other scientists to investigate colostrum at our colleges and universities. His experiences, both in the research field and in practical applications of colostrum, have increased our understanding of how valuable this natural remedy can be.

In this chapter, I'd like to share a few of the testimonies obtained from Dr. Plymate's book, ***Colostrum: Ancient Medicine in Our Time***. I want to say that testimonies and stories of healing, as presented here, are not to be considered claims that colostrum has brought about healing. Colostrum is a very valuable food, and we simply acknowledge it as such.

ANIMAL HEALING EXPERIENCES

In the case of a cow with an udder infection, a shot of processed, defatted colostrum (from another cow) in saline solution was given. The next day, the infection had cleared, showing that the immunity of one cow had been passed on to another. Not only did the infection heal, but the cow ate better and her coat grew healthier and improved in appearance.

Later, a friend showed up with her two children and a very sick cat that was limp and nearly lifeless. The cat was given a hypodermic shot of colostrum and was left to rest. Before long, one of the children said, "Mom, it's moving around!" They went out on the porch to see the cat. It actually got up and walked around before they took it home.

A neighbor had an old dog who could hardly get around. Stiff with arthritis, eyes dimmed with cataracts, he was just very old. Colostrum was put in his water dish and some extra was given to the neighbor to give the dog for a few days. In two or three days, the old dog was running around the yard like a puppy!

On another occasion, a banker in Iowa had a poodle with what the veterinarian said was a cancer on its eye—raw and irritated from the dog scratching it. The vet recommended putting the dog away, but they decided to try colostrum first. The dog was given colostrum in its food and water, and it was also sprayed on the bad eye several times a day. A week later, the dog's eye had healed.

Ten dogs, thirteen years old or older, were selected for a study on the effects of colostrum on aging processes. They received 20cc (a little under 1 tablespoon) each day in their drinking water. Their owners and the veterinarians participating in the study noticed improved ease of movement and greater agility. The sexual responsiveness of all five male dogs returned.

These stories are encouraging and interesting, but we find out the testimonies of people using colostrum are even more fascinating.

THE EARACHE THAT DISAPPEARED

The Plymate's little daughter developed a terrible earache one day, which increased in pressure until an abscess in the ear broke. Her father warmed some of the sterile liquid colostrum solution he had made up, put a little in her ear and she went to sleep. As the Plymate family proved over the years, colostrum was the best earache medicine they ever found.

FROM ARTHRITIS TO AMBITION

Dr. Plymate's mother happened to be one of the huge number of arthritis sufferers in the Midwest where they were living some years ago. When her feet began to swell, she started taking colostrum. The swelling left. She reported a feeling of well-being and told her son she felt "ambitious." I might say, that's the kind of well-being I mean when I say, "I feel wonderful!"

RECIPE FOR A CHRONICALLY PLUGGED-UP NOSE

A man whose nasal passages had been plugged for years received an eye dropper of colostrum solution in each nostril. After a while, he started sniffing, and his nose began to run from one side. He began blowing his nose on tissues and could hardly believe what was coming out. Then the other side of his nose began to run. The next day, he told a friend that he hadn't breathed so well in 25 years.

THE LOST WEDDING RING

A woman whose husband was taking colostrum decided to use some of it herself. She had arthritis in her hands with such pain and swelling in the knuckles that she hadn't had her wedding ring off in 15 years. As she was doing her dishes one day, she noticed her wedding ring was gone! The swelling in her knuckles had gone down so much that the ring apparently slipped off in the soapy dish water. She felt it was a small price to pay for getting rid of the pain and swelling in her knuckles.

A SURPRISING IMPROVEMENT IN THE PANCREAS

A nurse with diabetes, who was taking 56 units of insulin regularly, started taking colostrum orally and spraying a solution of colostrum on her leg to speed up the healing of ulcers on her legs. In three days, the ulcer developed a healthy scab. When she checked her blood sugar level, however, she found that her need for insulin had dropped considerably. In time, her insulin intake was reduced to 20 units.

Over the years, diabetics who use colostrum have reported improvement in two areas. First, they are finding their insulin need is less. Secondly, they are finding the toxicity level in their bodies is lowered.

THE LADY DECIDED TO GO HOME

Dr. Plymate's mother was taken to the hospital in great pain, which was diagnosed as a gallbladder attack. The doctor advised surgical removal as soon as possible and contacted a surgeon from a nearby town. She started taking colostrum at 3 pm and continued taking it, a total of several ounces. Around 11 pm that night, she had to go to the bathroom and kept going about five or six times. The colostrum appeared to stimulate and increase the ridding of toxins from her body. The next morning, the doctors who checked her before sending her to surgery found that the gallbladder area had softened up. One doctor recommended removing the gallbladder anyway, but the lady didn't go along with that opinion. The next morning, she decided to go home.

A CASE OF MIND-BODY IMPROVEMENT

A woman in her fifties, formerly married and divorced, was going through menopause while also suffering from a form of schizophrenia involving times of severe depression. She was taking a regular medication but agreed to try colostrum. The lady reported sleeping more soundly, an increased appetite and a greater sense of well-being. She stopped her medication and leads a nearly-normal life.

A DOCTOR DOCTORS HERSELF WITH COLOSTRUM

A woman medical doctor in her 70s, troubled with swollen legs, kidney problems and a breast tumor, decided to use colostrum. Before long, the swelling disappeared and the breast tumor first softened, then went away. As a result, this doctor began using colostrum in her practice to help other women with breast tumors. She also told other doctors.

RECOVERY FROM STOMACH SURGERY AND CHEMOTHERAPY

A man who had a cancerous part of his stomach removed was taking chemotherapy and also started taking colostrum. His blood count began to improve, his hair loss stopped and his hair began to grow back in again. He quit using the colostrum, and began losing hair again. He also began to get nauseated. He felt sure the colostrum had prevented the nausea and hair loss. This man is now doing very well.

HIGH BLOOD PRESSURE

When Dr. Bob Plymate found out he had high blood pressure (190/90), he began taking colostrum as well as garlic and parsley, which nutritionists often recommend for high blood pressure. Over a period of a year-and-a-half, not only did his blood pressure drop, but he began losing weight. He had been overweight and was grateful for the easy weight loss as well as the improved blood pressure.

CHAPTER 5

COLOSTRUM AND THE HEALING CRISIS

We have seen, in previous chapters, that nature cures, but sometimes she needs a helping hand. The immune system of man is truly a miraculous, almost unbelievably powerful system of protection. Yet, under the overwhelming pressures of life in high-technology, fast-lane cultures, diseases are emerging that are able to overwhelm, subvert or pervert the immune defenses that were originally designed to keep us healthy. The greatest challenge to the healing art in our time is to discover humane and effective responses to diseases such as AIDS, cancer, heart disease, lupus and other life-destructive conditions.

In this book, we are seeing how the rediscovery of an ancient food, like colostrum, can be a great help in tipping the scales of health in man's favor.

HERING'S LAW OF CURE

By modern standards, we find that health is measured by the absence of symptoms. The deceptiveness of this standard is immediately seen when the American Cancer Society tells us that some cancers take as long as 20 years to develop. This means that only after 20 years do symptoms begin to manifest. Yet, the disease was forming in the body undetected all that time. The absence of symptoms doesn't mean we are well.

Because of this health standard, based on detectable symptoms, abuse of the body is socially and politically tolerated as long as symptoms have not yet appeared. So, we find that smoking, alcohol abuse, drug addiction, use of food adulterated by harmful chemicals, obesity and other harmful activities and conditions are allowed and condoned in our society even though we know there are disease consequences to all of them. Much of today's disease is earned by deliberate neglect of nature's laws of health.

The emphasis in health care, according to this way of thinking, is to suppress symptoms. Doctors and hospitals are now beginning to see that without teaching their patients how to live a healthy lifestyle, they will return. People who don't learn from their mistakes repeat them.

Symptoms are signals from mother nature that something in the patient's body or life or both is seriously out of balance. The right thing to do, then, is not to suppress the symptom but to discover its cause and correct the problem.

Sometime in the late 1800s, the European homeopath, Constantine Hering, made a remarkable set of observations that led to what we know as Hering's law. This law states, "All cure starts from the head down, from the inside out, and in reverse order as symptoms first appeared." This law forms the basis on which much of the natural healing art rests.

I use Hering's law constantly in my practice to guide and shape my work with patients. It accurately describes the healing process in man when we work with nature instead of against it.

We find that natural healing requires three preconditions for the reversal of disease. First, we must stop doing those things that break down the body, things that helped bring on the disease and keep it going. Second, we need to make sure all elimination channels—bowel, kidneys, skin, lungs and bronchials—are working as well as possible so we can get rid of toxic accumulations and old catarrh. Third, we need to adopt a health-building food regimen that includes whole, pure and natural foods. These foods must be varied from day to day to make sure we are meeting our whole body's nutritional needs.

When we have met these preconditions, we see Hering's law go to work.

The first part of Hering's law says, "All cure starts from the head down." As we strengthen the body and provide the proper balance of whole, pure and natural foods, the brain centers that regulate all organs, glands and tissues in the body begin to raise the metabolic rate and energy level until it reaches a level at which catarrh and toxins begin to discharge through the body's elimination channels and sometimes through other orifices of the body.

The second part of Hering's law is that cure comes from "the inside out." The discharging and elimination of long-accumulated metabolic wastes, heavy metals, catarrh, drug residues, nicotine and tar and other undesirable substances is a cleansing from the body of all the locked-in waste and debris that were suppressing the immune system and feeding the disease.

Third, Hering's law predicts that old symptoms will be re-experienced, starting with the most recent symptoms first. This takes place "in reverse order as symptoms first appeared." This is the way nature reverses disease processes in the body, if we do not hinder by suppressing the symptoms or discharges. Symptoms from the most recent problems to the most distant, sometimes going back decades in a person's life, may be experienced, although not necessarily in one single episode.

THE HEALING CRISIS

The healing crisis is the culmination of Hering's law. It differs from a disease crisis in that it usually begins when a person is feeling "on top of the world." On the other hand, a disease crisis is usually experienced after a series of warning signs, including chronic fatigue and catarrhal problems.

A person may have several healing crises in the course of a year or even several years, each occurring after a period of improving health and increasing strength, involving the three preconditions to all natural healing—stop breaking down, improve elimination and the use of whole, pure and natural foods.

A healing crisis can be a very difficult process to endure, but it should be warmly welcomed as a much preferred option over continuing with a disease. It also shows that your attempts to build up strength and health are working. If a healing crisis does not take place in some reasonable time frame, such as a year, then a person should go over his diet regimen, exercise and other health-building steps with a doctor who knows natural healing.

Symptoms signaling the onset of a healing crisis may include nausea, vomiting, diarrhea, headaches, fever, chills, muscle aches, itching, coughing and possibly discharges from one or more orifices of the body. Onset is often sudden and very severe the first day, and less severe in the following days. A healing crisis usually lasts from three to five days, seldom longer.

During the crisis, juices and broths may be taken, especially my potato peeling broth, as follows: Simmer peelings from two potatoes, cut 1/4-inch deep, in three cups of water for 15 minutes. Strain and drink. Vegetable broth powder may be added for flavor, or other vegetables chopped fine, such as onion, carrots, celery and so forth. This broth is high in potassium, which helps to neutralize the acids released during a healing crisis.

After the healing crisis is over, new tissue begins to come in to replace the old. This is what we have worked for—a restoration of tissue integrity.

COLOSTRUM AND THE HEALING CRISIS

Colostrum aids in the development of a healing crisis in several ways. Before the healing crisis takes place, the elimination channels are often underactive and the immune system may be suppressed. Colostrum provides substantial aid to both systems.

One of the immunoglobulins in colostrum protects the bowel wall and neutralizes dangerous toxins in the bowel. Colostrum feeds and encourages the growth of the beneficial acidophilus bacteria in the bowel, which, in turn, suppresses unfavorable bacteria populations such as E. coli and yeast infections such as Candida. This improves bowel efficiency in preparation for the crisis.

Immune system support from colostrum is provided in many ways. Immunoglobulins and antibodies in colostrum may assist in destroying bacteria and viruses contributing to the problem. A proline-rich polypeptide in colostrum stimulates an underactive immune system. Nucleotides and vitamins are supplied for immune system support, while accessory factors like peroxidase, lactoferrin and polysaccharides also strengthen immunity. Adenosine monophosphate helps raise the energy level.

In other words, colostrum assists in building up the two key systems that do most of the work during a healing crisis. Additionally, colostrum contains a growth factor that will speed up the replacement of disease-damaged tissue after the healing crisis.

The great advantage of colostrum is that it is a food, not a drug or medicine. No adverse effects have been noted, nor is overdose a danger. Colostrum was designed by nature to be gentle enough for baby animals to take, yet strong enough to protect them from a number of very dangerous diseases.

Colostrum is a tremendous aid and benefit in working toward a healing crisis, as well as in building new tissue afterward.

CHAPTER **6**

DR. JENSEN'S PERSONAL TESTIMONY

In early February 1991, I flew to Arizona to have my teeth worked on by my dentist. He wanted to cut back my gums to take care of an infection from a periodontal condition. I decided to go on a week of juice fasting to see if I could take care of the infection that way, so I bought juices in Phoenix and gave it a try. It was a very hectic time, because I had so much to do.

My dentist worked on my teeth for three days. With all the pounding, scraping, grinding and everything else, it took a lot out of me. He would have done the work over a longer period of time, but I said, "Let's get it over with so I can get back to my work at the Ranch." Then I drove 200 miles to have my jaw adjusted by a chiropractor who specializes in that kind of work.

When I returned home, I didn't feel that anything in particular was wrong. I don't recall doing anything to my back, but then I noticed I couldn't bend over to tie my shoes. It seemed like my back just went out, and I couldn't move it.

Of course, being a chiropractor myself, I've encountered people whose backs went out even bending over to pick up a handkerchief. They claimed it was serious, and I accepted it as such.

Starting right away, I had adjustments from a very good chiropractor and did everything I should for that kind of back problem. However, there were very quick twitches in my back that would almost bring me down to the floor if I touched that place or moved in a certain way. Any quick movements would really throw me. I knew I had a problem, but I didn't realize it was not a normal problem, as I will explain.

I went back to work. I had a run-in with one of the employees, telling him not to talk to other employees because he was interfering with their work. I kind of blew my stack. When I left the room, my back was a lot worse. That should have given me a clue that the problem wasn't due to twisting or turning.

Under the impact of emotional stress, the back became much worse. As I thought about it, iridology had shown for years that the right side of my back should have been giving me trouble, but it wasn't. I always had trouble with the left side of my back—until this most recent problem. Now I was having a right back problem.

I started analyzing everything. I had even fasted and we'd been having the nicest weather, so I couldn't blame my physical condition on the weather. I blamed the recession. I blamed the war with Iraq. I blamed my financial situation. I blamed the employees. I blamed the stress of preparing for an important trip. I blamed the emotional strain from all these things.

Well, I went through all this, then decided to cut things off a bit, slow the tempo and give myself a little rest.

One night I went into a serious sweat. I sweated like I never had before, and it lasted from an hour to an hour-and-a-half. I began having active bowel eliminations, better than I'd had in years.

WHY DID THIS HAPPEN?

I had forgotten or possibly just pushed to one side of my mind the fact that I'd been taking a colostrum product throughout this whole episode. I had been taking it before I went to Arizona, taking it during my time there, and taking it after I returned home. This product had apparently built up my strength and resistance and was able to bring on a healing crisis.

The next morning, after my night sweat, I had no more back problem.

I definitely feel I had an infection—I believe in the prostate gland. I haven't had a single twitch since that time. As carefully as I could, I twisted my back this way and that way, without even the smallest sign of pain. I have a slight ache like that of a boil receding, but as I'm writing this, I feel the best I've felt in weeks.

What happened to me, I believe, is the same thing I encourage my patients to look for—the reversal process and a healing crisis. I believe that taking my nutritional supplement raised the strength and metabolic level of my body to a healing crisis—getting rid of latent and tissue-stored toxins by starting a discharge activity.

Looking back, I recall several types of discharges. My ears were discharging. I had a sore throat. The lymph glands on the right side of my neck were swollen. I was bringing up an excessive amount of catarrh, with a constant nasal discharge and some coughing. Every year I've had a little coughing problem.

Last year, I had my doctor take care of a lung condition instead of changing my diet or going on a little juice fast. Possibly the condition was suppressed instead of being cleared up. I had too much work to do to take the time to take care of the problem by natural reversal.

This time I believe I had a healing crisis with the kind of elimination I needed to take care of the problem. It was a fever that brought on such heavy perspiration. Hippocrates said, "Give me the spirit of a fever, and I'll cure any disease."

I didn't realize I was having a healing crisis. I feel I had an infection, probably a low-grade flu that affected everything in my body from my teeth and gums to the lymph glands, bronchial tubes, prostate, throat and nose. While my bowels were good during the healing crisis, they are better now than they've ever been through all of this, another indication of a healing crisis.

I don't know why I didn't see this while it was taking place, but I'm convinced that my healing crisis was brought on by my food supplement with the colostrum in it.

IT'S A PERSONAL THING

Now I see how my emotional stress lowered my immunity, but the colostrum food supplement brought it back up. Emotional stress brought on the back problem, the prostate infection, the bronchial inflammation and all my catarrhal problems. I see how this all comes together now.

Every person who is going through physical problems, possibly even stress-related like my recent problems, must be told that with a better body, a stronger body, things would change. They must know that the conditions in their body, the symptoms they have experienced in the past, would begin to reverse. They would begin to retrace the old problems and conditions as their body grows stronger. The fatigue and tiredness would diminish as the energy and strength are restored. This is the way to a healing crisis.

THE HEALING CRISIS AND THE REVERSAL PROCESS

As I mentioned before, Hering's law says, "All cure comes from the head down, the inside out and in reverse order as symptoms first appeared." This is the natural law that points to the healing crisis. This is nature's way of healing.

We have to go through the healing crisis to get rid of all the catarrh, phlegm, metabolic wastes and other toxic materials held in the inherently weak tissues of the body, materials that hinder the healing and tissue-replacement process until they are gotten rid of. We have to get rid of the old so the new can come in. That happens when we've built a better body with better foods—and I've had it demonstrated to me. I feel the results of my healing crisis are just out of this world!

I know a man who had a cyst on his prostate gland and had to take care of it. He started taking colostrum. A week later, he was in agony. He was going through the worst pain he had ever been through in his life. Despite his misery, he recognized the colostrum was building up his strength and resistance. He knew he had to get the intestinal tract taken care of, which is one of colostrum's strong points. It helps develop a friendly bowel flora.

He spent a week in agony, and I can sympathize with him. I've had my week of agony and know what it's like. I can take a lot of pain, but never have I experienced pain as badly as during this past February.

After a week of nearly intolerable pain, this man developed a large boil on his buttock—almost as big as a lemon—and it began to drain. The draining gave him relief from his painful prostate cyst. By the time the boil finished draining and began to heal, he was free of prostate symptoms. He has had no trouble since that time. He is feeling better than ever before.

THE HEALING CRISIS—A WORTHWHILE GOAL

I tell my patients they are working toward their healing crisis as a worthwhile goal. I've worked with many people, helping them toward a healing crisis. But the average lifestyle of people these days doesn't bring on a healing crisis very fast.

You have to work at building the best body possible, through a balanced food regimen, exercise and healthful living habits. I usually tell my patients not to expect a healing crisis in less than a year.

The truth is, if you take care of the bowel, everything else improves. I discovered this many years ago when I developed my 7-day Tissue Cleansing Program. Whenever people took my bowel cleansing program, every organ in their bodies improved.

Now I believe if we impress upon a person that they will end up with the best body possible, they will be happy to work toward a healing crisis. I don't believe that people who aren't willing to be changed can be helped. I don't believe anything will help an alcoholic who wants to keep drinking. I don't believe it will help a smoker who wants to keep smoking. It can't even be for a junk food junkie who won't give up his habit.

The healing crisis is for a person who wants to get rid of his troubles and get started on a right way of living and keep it up for the rest of his life. I went through the healing crisis despite all the work I was doing. I felt like I was able to handle it.

What is wonderful is to know that nature has provided a remedy that can work on a person even in his 60s, 70s and 80s to reverse disease and build a greater sense of well-being.

CHAPTER 7

CONCLUDING THOUGHTS ON COLOSTRUM

Looking back over my 60 years or so serving in the healing arts, I feel one of my greatest strengths has been discovering products, processes and programs that truly assist in reversing the pathways of a significant number of chronic diseases. I can't tell you how many patients have come to my sanitariums "as a last resort," after their doctors had given up on them. Many of them recovered completely and have remained free of the disease that originally brought them to me. I only wanted to see them get well—and many did.

At various times I have relied upon such foods as liquid chlorophyll for cleansing the body, protomorphogens for strengthening organs or glands, high RNA foods for rebuilding tissue, dried goat whey (Whex) to restore sodium to the joints and gastrointestinal system, herbs for cleansing the body and taking care of symptoms, chlorella for speeding up the rate of healing and detoxification, honey bee pollen to build the blood and assist many metabolic processes, aloe vera for external and internal problems and many other fine products. I have used these supplements together with a balanced food regimen to eliminate chemical shortages in the body and to stimulate a reversal of disease.

I have used processes such as diets, fasting, exercise, Kneipp baths, color therapy, positive affirmations, colonics, personology and bowel management to help my patients learn to leave their diseases behind and live in a new day.

By combining a balanced food regimen with selected nutritional supplements and health-building processes, I have developed programs that have been particularly effective for many individuals.

In other words, I have spent most of my life learning everything I could to help you avoid or reverse disease, find a healthy lifestyle and live a long and wonderful life.

Each time I came across a disease-reversing and health-building product or process, I became excited, not because I expected to become rich or famous, but because I would be able to help more people—like you, for example.

I have never claimed any product, process or program to be a "cure-all." In fact, I have never claimed to cure anybody of anything. What I believe is that nature cures, but sometimes she needs a helping hand.

Foods, food supplements, processes like bowel cleansing and programs like weight reduction are only effective in preventing (or reversing) disease and in building health to the degree that they work in harmony with the body's own natural functions. For example, certain herbs and food supplements like chlorella and aloe vera tend to stimulate detoxification of tissues, a function normally provided by the lymph system and blood in cooperation with the liver and with metabolic rate controls in the brain and endocrine system. In other words, they cooperate with and strengthen natural systems in the body. When toxic materials imbedded in the inherently weak tissues are pried loose, flushed into the lymph and eliminated from the body, repairing and rebuilding can begin. Cleansing of tissues must come before repair can take place.

ANOTHER MASTER PRODUCT

Special foods and food supplements that accomplish some especially important job in the body may be called *master products*—high-level health enhancers.

Colostrum is such a product, and once again, I am excited to be able to share a wonderful discovery with my friends and readers.

I am not saying I discovered colostrum, or that I am the first to realize its health benefits. But, I may be the first one to realize the importance and potential power of colostrum in protecting the bowel and thereby reducing the flow of bowel toxins into the blood and lymph, perhaps the most dangerous and most underestimated source of disease in the body. The average bowel is literally a polluted cesspool of decomposing food wastes, chemical food additives, drug residues, bacteria, viruses, fungi, metabolic waste products of microorganisms, chemicals from treated water supplies and reactive processed foods like bleached white flour, refined sugar and overheated fats and oils.

Colostrum, by means of its active immune factors, protects the bowel from harm due to dangerous internal microorganisms, their toxic by-products and other potentially damaging substances.

Basically, by helping protect the bowel, colostrum frees the immune system to be more active in protecting the rest of the body from diseases and harmful bacteria, viruses and other harmful substances.

Colostrum contains several different immune factors, including leukocytes capable of producing interferon (which protects cells from viral destruction), hormones—including an insulin-like hormone (which helps cells use blood sugar), a proline-containing polypeptide (which helps normalize immunity), another polypeptide that promotes tissue repair, seven nucleotides (molecules that make up nucleic acids) and three immunoglobulins (IgG, IgA and IgM). I have listed the contents of colostrum in a previous chapter.

Ig is short for immunoglobulin, and the three classes of immuno-globulins in colostrum from cows are the same classes found in humans—IgG, IgA and IgM. Each immunoglobulin can be varied to create a great variety of antibodies, so that no matter what kind of antigen enters the body, an antibody can be formed to destroy it from one of the classes.

Each immunoglobulin class has a job to do in protecting the body. Secretory (sIgA) and IgA are found in body secretions like milk, saliva, tears and mucus. They are prevalent throughout the gastrointestinal tract, including the mouth and throat. IgA antibodies will attack any bacteria, virus or fungus that tries to enter the body. If one of these antigens succeeds in entering the body, we have two classes of immunoglobulins that form antibodies that circulate in the blood and lymph. IgG antibodies are very effective in neutralizing toxins, including the highly-toxic wastes of some bacteria and viruses. IgM antibodies destroy harmful bacteria.

Immunoglobulins are made of chains of amino acids, the same building blocks of which all proteins are made. IgG is made up of two light chains of about 220 amino acids and two heavy chains of about 440 amino acids. IgM is much bigger than IgG, and has 20 chains, 10 light and 10 heavy. The chains are linked together with sulfur atoms.

In a child or adult, antibodies are formed in lymph nodes, the spleen and other lymph tissue, as well as by plasma cells in the blood and by lymphocytes. But, as we have seen, antibodies also come from the immunoglobulins in colostrum, and they have the same protective effect as those made in our own bodies.

OTHER IMMUNE BUILDING FOODS

I have studied the edible alga chlorella pyrenoidosa (the best of many types of chlorella algae) for many years now, and I use it often with patients whose immune systems are rundown. Chlorella grows in nutrient-rich water at a faster rate than any other known vegetation, and the growth factor that makes this possible stimulates healing in humans and animals with injuries or disease-damaged tissue. Chlorella contains ingredients that stimulate cellular immunity and protect against bacteria like E. coli. I believe in the benefits of chlorella very much.

But, as far as I know, processed colostrum from cows is the highest source of immunoglobulins. While cows' milk is only 10% protein, cows' colostrum is 20% protein, and 55% of this is immunoglobulins which are active in destroying disease-producing microbes. I feel that this immunity-building food has been recognized at a time when it is needed the most.

Modern life, poor food habits and unhealthy lifestyles are suppressing and handicapping our immune system function until more people are vulnerable to dangerous diseases and ailments than ever before in the history of man. I feel that the new concentrated colostrum is just what we need at this time in history.

Colostrum is a food, not a drug, so there are no undesirable side effects, cumulative effects or time-bomb effects. There are enzymes present in the colostrum that prevent its immunoglobulins from being digested, so that it immediately goes to work in the bowel, reducing toxicity and protecting against undesirable bowel flora.

TWO KINDS OF IMMUNITY

There are two main kinds of immunity in the body and they work together to protect us from disease or harm from foreign substances. They are cellular immunity and humoral immunity. Antibodies are part of the humoral immunity system because they circulate constantly through the body. Lymphocytes and granulocytes are part of cellular immunity, and I will explain how they work together.

Most of what we know about antibodies has been learned in the past twenty-five years. When a dangerous microbe enters into the body, antibodies are produced to respond to it. There are molecular "keys" on the surface of the antibody that are designed to fit into molecular "keyholes" on the surface of the microbe. The antibody is only a tiny bit of protein, one-thousandth the size of an average bacteria, but it sticks to a microbe like glue and cannot be shaken off.

Antibodies can render a toxin harmless, but they don't directly destroy bacteria. Instead, they begin a series of steps where the bacteria are destroyed.

The next step after an antibody locks onto a bacteria is that the antibody changes its shape to attract circulating chemical proteins called "complement." There are 20 parts to complement, and they are perfectly safe (inactivated) while they circulate in the blood, but when they begin to stick together with an antibody on the back of a bacteria, an unusual thing happens.

As each of the 20 members of complement protein attach to the antibody and bacteria, chemicals are released on the surface of the bacteria that make a hole in its cell wall. This happens in the space of tenths of a second. The damaged bacteria is then consumed by white blood cells of any of a variety of kinds, such as macrophages or granulocytes.

While bacteria and fungi can be eliminated this way, viruses and parasites have to be removed in another way. Viruses and parasites get inside cells. Messenger lymphocytes which have noted a viral or parasitic infection go to the nearest lymph node and "touch" a cell called a T-cell ("T" indicates that it has been activated by the thymus gland). The T-cell is then transformed into what is called a "Killer-T-cell," which leaves the lymph node and destroys the virus-infected cells. Killer T-cells are able to "lock onto" infected cells the way antibodies "lock onto" bacteria and fungi. Then they release a chemical poison that destroys the infected cell and the virus it contains.

Antibodies also destroy many viruses, but there are some they can't destroy. And AIDS, the disease known as autoimmune deficiency syndrome, actually infects the immune system itself, destroying the components of our immunity that would normally destroy the virus that causes AIDS.

There is much more to immunity than I have described here, but this will give you an idea of how important the immune system is, and why we should support and protect it by using colostrum regularly.

Colostrum not only aids humoral immunity but cellular immunity as well, stimulating production of at least one type of lymphocyte.

THE POTENTIAL OF COLOSTRUM

Studies with cow colostrum have shown that people who take two teaspoons of it every day experience an improved quality of life. They develop more "get-up-and-go" than they have had in years. I believe this is because their immune systems are getting much needed support and because tissue repair is being enhanced.

These days, our immune systems are being constantly overworked. We need to take care of them, and the best product for doing this is colostrum, in my opinion.

I am personally excited about the great potential for improved resistance to disease, improved quality of life and increased longevity in those who begin to use colostrum regularly.

AFTERTHOUGHTS

I have no doubt that there will soon be many colostrum products introduced in health food stores after this book has circulated a while throughout its popular audience, and people start talking about the potential of this unusual food supplement.

You should be warned that most of them will not be of the highest quality. Many will be just dried whey products with little power or benefit. **You must understand that not all cows provide the kind of colostrum** that produces the kinds of benefits described in this book.

The colostrum I use—and believe in so strongly—comes from selected, pre-tested, disease-free, registered, grade-A dairy cows that have given birth to at least three calves. These are the qualities required to bring out the greatest amount of immune factors in colostrum, the factors that can mean so much in restoring or building health.

Although many individuals are allergic to or intolerant of milk and milk products, I must tell you that colostrum is not milk and it doesn't contain the same combination of ingredients. **There have been no reported cases of allergic reaction to colostrum.**

BIBLIOGRAPHY FOR FURTHER STUDY

Acosta-Altamirano, G., *et al.* (1987), "Antiamoebic Properties of Human Colostrum," ***Advances in Experimental Medicine and Biology, 216B,*** pp. 1347-1352.

Ballard, F. John and Francis, Geoffrey L. (1983), "Effects of Anabolic Agents on Protein Breakdown in L6 Myoblasts," ***Journal of Biochemistry, 210,*** pp. 243-249. (Describes how protein breakdown in tissue due to injury is inhibited by several anabolic agents including an insulin-like substance in bovine colostrum.)

Ballard, F. John; Nield, M.K.; Francis, Geofrey L., *et al.* (1982), "The Relationship Between the Insulin Content and Inhibitory Effects of Bovine Colostrum on Protein Breakdown in Cultured Cells," ***Journal of Cellular Physiology, 110,*** pp. 249-254. (Insulin-like ingredient in bovine colostrum slows protein breakdown in several cell lines. Protein breakdown was also slowed by addition of colostrum to a cell line known to be unresponsive to insulin, indicating the presence of non-insulin growth factors in bovine colostrum.)

Bouda, J., *et al.*, (1987), "Trypsin Inhibitor Activity in the Colostrum of Cows," ***Veterinarni Medicina,*** Vol. ***32***, No. ***3***, pp. 135-144. (Greatest trypsin activity was in the colostrum of the first milking after calving.)

Bouda, J., *et al.*, (1980), "Vitamin A and Carotene Metabolism in Cows and Their Calves Fed from Buckets," ***Acta Veterinaria Brno.***, Vol. ***49***, Nos. ***1-2***, pp. 45-52. (Vitamin A in bovine colostrum is ten times the amount in serum. Vitamin A assists in restoring and revitalizing the thymus gland.)

Bouda, J., *et al.*, (1980), "Vitamins E and C in the Blood Plasma of Cows and Their Calves Fed from Buckets," ***Acta Veterinaria Brno.***, Vol. ***49***, Nos. ***1-2***, pp. 53-58. (Vitamin E is 2.5 times greater in bovine colostrum than in milk. It helps protect the vitamin A and other ingredients from oxidation.)

Brandtzaeg, Per, (1983), "The Secretory Immune System of Lactating Human Mammary Glands Compared with Other Exocrine Organs," ***Annals of New York Academy of Sciences, 409***, pp. 353-378. (Immune factors present in the mother are transmitted to the infant until its immune system is operative. Immunoglobulins are able to neutralize the most harmful bacteria, viruses and yeasts.)

Buescher, E.S. and McIlheran, S.M., (1988), "Antioxidant Properties of Human Colostrum," ***Pediatric Research,*** Vol. ***24***, No. ***1***, pp. 14-19.

Crago, Sylvia S. and Mestecky, Jiri, (1983), "Immunoinhibitory Elements in Human Colostrum," ***Survey of Immunol. Res.***, Vol. ***2***, No. ***2***, pp. 164-169. (A protein substance was found in colostrum which inhibits the overproduction of lymphocytes stimulated by antigens and mitogens and may reduce symptoms associated with allergic reactions.)

Cruz, Jose R., *et al.*, (1983), "Specific Immune Response in Human Milk to Oral Immunization with Food Protein," ***Annals of N.Y. Academy of Sciences, 409***, pp. 808-809. (Immune factors from blood serum are added to mammary secretions.)

Dluholucky, S., *et al.*, (1980), "Antimicrobial Activity of Colostrum after Administering Killed Escherichia Coli 011 Vaccine Orally to Expectant Mothers," ***Archives of Diseases in Childhood, 55***, pp. 458-460. (Naturally-developed immune factors from mucosal sources that enter blood serum may become concentrated in expectant mothers' mammary glands.)

Ebina, T., *et al.*, (1983), "Prevention of Rotavirus Infection by Cow Colostrum Containing Antibody Against Human Rotavirus," ***The Lancet***, Vol. ***29***, No. ***2***, pp. 1029-1030. (Japanese researchers exposed cattle to oral doses of rotavirus which causes severe diarrhea and bowel inflammation in humans. Colostrum from these cows contained antibodies which, when fed to humans, prevented them from getting rotavirus.)

Eldridge, John H., *et al.* (1983), "Peyer's Patches Accessory Cells Bear I-1," ***Annals of N.Y. Academy of Sciences, 409***, pp. 819-821. (Groups of cells in the mucosa of the intestinal tract, known as Peyer's Patches produce immune factors.)

Francis, Geoffrey L.; Upton, Faye M.; Ballard, F. John, *et al.*, (1988), "Insulin-Like Growth Factors 1 and 2 in Bovine Colostrum," ***Journal of Biochemistry, 251***, pp. 95-103. (Two growth factors similar to insulin were purified from bovine colostrum and found to be very similar to corresponding human growth factors. In this experiment protein synthesis was increased and protein breakdown was reduced by administration of the bovine colostrum extracts.)

Francis, Geoffrey L., *et al.*, (1986), "Purification and Partial Sequence Analysis of Insulin-Like Growth Factor 1 from Bovine Colostrum," ***Biochemical Journal, 233(1)***, pp. 207-213.

Frankenne, F., *et al.*, (1989), "Purification and Characterization of Insulin-Like Growth Factor 1 from Cow Colostrum," ***Biochemical Society Transactions***, Vol. ***17***, No. ***3***, p. 602.

Gil, Angel and Sanchez-Medina, Fermin, (1981), "Acid Soluble Nucleotides of Cow's, Goat's and Sheep's Milk at Different Stages of Lactation," ***Journal of Dairy Research***, Vol. ***48***, No. ***1***, pp. 35-41. (Bovine colostrum was found to contain seven different nucleotides.)

Hanson, *et al.*, (1983), "Mucosal Immunity," ***Annals of N.Y. Academy of Sciences, 409***, 15ff. (The immune system produces immunoglobulins, antibodies, leukocytes, macrophages, interferon and other factors for defending the body. Immune factors from specialized cell groups in the bronchials and bowel travel away from their sources to coat the passages of the lungs and bowels and destroy antigens, allergens and pathogens. Immune factors from colostrum other than immunoglobulins blocked attachment of many types of bacteria to mucous membranes. Oligosaccharides—big sugar molecules—from colostrum blocked attached of *Streptococcus* *pneumonococci*, a major cause of lung inflammations and middle ear infections.)

Ho, P.C. and Lawton, John W.M., (1978), "Human Colostral Cells: Phagocytosis and Killing of E. Coli and C. Albicans," ***The Journal of Pediatrics***, Vol. ***93***, No. ***6***, pp. 910-915. (Ho and Lawton at the Queen Mary Hospital in Hong Kong showed that colostrum leukocytes were effective against the bacteria *E. coli* and the yeast *Candida albicans*.)

Janusz, M., *et al.*, (1987), "Immunoregulatory Properties of Synthetic Peptides, Fragments of a Proline-Rich Polypeptide from Bovine Colostrum," ***Molecular Immunology***, Vol ***24***, No. ***10***, pp. 1029-1031. (A nonapeptide fragment was isolated from the chymotryptic digest of PRP. The nonapeptide showed biological activity similar to PRP.)

Julius, Michael H., Janusz, Maria and Lisowski, Jozef, (1988), "A Colostral Protein that Induces the Growth and Differentiation of Resting B Lymphocytes," ***Journal of Immunology***, Vol. ***140***, No. **5**, pp. 1366-1371.

Juto, P., (1985), "Human Milk Stimulates B-Cell Function," ***Archives of Disease in Childhood***, Vol. ***60***, No. ***7***, pp. 610-613. (Mature breast milk as well as filtered, defatted, cell-free colostrum enhanced B-cell proliferation and antibody secretion but the same activities were not observed in milk-substitute formula. This partly explains why breast-fed babies are healthier.)

Kim, K., *et al.*, (1985), "In Vitro and In Vitro Neutralizing Activity of Human Colostrum and Milk Against Purified Toxins A and B of Clostridium Difficile," ***Journal of Infectious Diseases***, Vol. ***150***, No. ***1***, pp. 57-61. (Substances from colostrum neutralize the two main toxins of the clostridium bacteria which are believed to cause illness.)

Klagsbrun, M., (1978), "Human Milk Stimulates DNA Synthesis and Cellular Proliferation in Cultured Fibroblasts," ***Proceedings of the National Academy of Sciences, 75***, pp. 5057-5061. (Growth factors in milk showed 100 times the potency of calf serum when tested on fibroblasts.)

Klagsbrun, M., (1980), "Bovine Colostrum Supports the Serum-Free Proliferation of Epithelial Cells but not of Fibroblasts in Long-Term Culture," ***Journal of Cellular Biology, 84***, pp. 808-814.

Kuhl, S., *et al.*, (1978), "Human Colostral Cytotoxicity: Antibody-Dependent Cellular Cytotoxicity Against Herpes Simplex Viral-Infected Cells Mediated by Colostral Cells," ***Journal of Clinical Laboratory Immunology, 1***, pp. 221-224. (Colostral cells along with antibody were found to destroy *herpes simplex*-infected cells.)

Lawton, J.W.M., *et al.*, (1979), "Interferon Synthesis by Human Colostral Leukocytes," ***Archives of Diseases in Childhood, 54***, pp. 127-130. (Exposure of colostrum leukocytes to certain mitogens stimulated production of interferon, the substance that slows or prevents viral growth.)

Ley, Beth M., (1990), ***Colostrum: Nature's Gift to the Immune System***, published by BL Productions.

McGhee, Jerry R., (1983), "Introductory Remarks," New York Academy of Sciences Conference on Secretory Immunity in 1982, as reported in ***Annals of the NY Academy of Sciences, 409***, p. xiii.

McClead, Richard, *et al.*, (1982), "Resistance of Bovine Anti-Cholera Toxin IgGl (Anti-CT) to *In Vitro* and *In Vivo* Proteolosis," ***Pediatric Research***, Vol ***6***, No. ***4***, p. 227. (Colostrum from cows exposed to cholera contained IgG antibodies which protected against that type of cholera.)

Majumdar, Anis S., *et al.*, (1982), "Protective Properties of Anticholera Antibodies in Human Colostrum," ***Infection and Immunology***, Vol. ***36***, No. ***3***, pp. 962-965. (Mothers in India exposed to cholera passed on protective antibodies to their newborns which prevented them from getting the disease.)

Michaels, R.H., (1965), "Studies of Antiviral Factors in Human Milk and Serum," ***Journal of Immunology, 94***, pp. 262-268. (Neutralizing factors for the Coxsackie and Echo viruses were found in colostrum.)

Moldoveanu, Zina, *et al.*, (1983), "Antibacterial Properties of Milk: IgA—Peroxidase Lactoferrin Interactions," ***Annals of***

NY Academy of Sciences, 409, pp. 848-850. (Combination of peroxidase, lactoferrin and IgA in colostrum produce strong antibacterial effect.)

Moro, I., *et al.*, (1985), "Natural Killer Cells in Human Colostrum," ***Cellular Immunology, 93(2)***, pp. 467-474. (Approximately 0.5% of colostral cells were identified as natural killer cells of two morphological types.)

Morris, J.A., *et al.*, (1980), "Passive Protection of Lambs Against Enteropathogenic Escherichia Coli: Role of Antiobodies in Serum and Colostrum of Dams Vaccinated with K99 Antigen," ***Journal of Medical Microbiology***, Vol. ***13***, No. ***2***, pp. 265-271. (Mother sheep and cows given doses of *E. coli* orally developed antibodies for *E. coli* in their colostrum. When nursing offspring were then dosed with *E. coli*, immune factors from the mothers' colostrum prevented the *E. coli* from attaching to the bowel wall and protection resulted.)

Oda, Shinnichi, *et al.*, (1989), "Insulin-Like Growth Factor 1, GH, Insulin and Glucagon Concentrations in Bovine Colostrum and in Plasma of Dairy Cows and Neonatal Calves Around Parturition," ***Comparative Biochemical Physiology, A: Comparative Physiology***, Vol. ***94A***, No. ***4***, pp. 805-808.

Ogra, Pearay, *et al.*, (1983), "Colostrum Derived Immunity and Maternal Neonatal Interaction," ***Annals of NY Academy of Sciences, 409***, pp. 82-92. (Peyer's patches are found throughout the intestinal tract and groups of immunoactive cells like them are found in the bronchial mucosa. Both the intestinal and bronchial immunoactive cell groups respond to allergens, antigens and pathogens by neutralizing or destroying them. In newborns, these special cell groups are not immediately operative but protection is provided by a variety of immune factors from the mother's colostrum. Antibodies found in colostrum protect against *E. coli, Salmonella, Shigella, V. cholera, Bacteriodes fragilis, Streptococcus pneumoniae, Bordtella pertussis, Clostridium diptheriae, Clostridium tetani* and *Streptococcus mutans*. Colostrum also contains antibodies against *Candida albicans*.)

Ott, V.D. and Marushko, T.L., (1985), "Immunobiological Role of Human Colostrum and Milk," ***Pediatriia*** (USSR), ***10***, pp. 72-75.

Palmer, E.L., *et al.*, (1980), "Antiviral Activity of Colostrum and Serum Immunoglobulins A and G," ***Journal of Medical Virology***, ***5***, pp. 123-129. (Colostrum has enteric virus secretory antibody that acts against viruses excreted from the bowel. A wide range of antiviral factors were acknowledged to be present in colostrum and milk. This research was done at the prestigious Center for Disease Control in Atlanta, Georgia.)

Paul, P.S., *et al.*, (1983), "Persistence of Passively Acquired Antibodies to Hemaglutinating Encephalomyelitis Virus in Swine," ***American Journal of Veterinary Research***, Vol. ***45***, No. ***5***, pp. 932-934. (Colostrum antibodies were effective against a severe virus in pigs.)

Paulik, S., *et al.*, (1985), "Lysozyme in the Colostrum and Blood of Calves of Dairy Cows," ***Veterinarni Medicina*** (Poland, Vol. ***30***, No. ***1***, pp. 21-28. (Lysozyme is the enzyme present in egg white, tears, saliva and other body fluids that kills certain bacteria by dissolving their cell walls.)

Plymate, Robert, (1982), ***Colostrum: Ancient Medicine for Our Time***, published by Bobra Publishing, Rogers, Arkansas.

Rouse, B.T., *et al.*, (1976), "Antibody-Dependent Cell-Mediated Cytotoxicity in Cows: Comparison of Effector Cell Activity Against Heterologous Erythrocyte and Herpes-Virus-Infected Bovine Target Cells," ***Infection and Immunity, 13***, p. 1433. (Bovine colostral cells with antibody were able to kill cells infected with *herpes simplex*.)

Sabin, Albert B., (1950), "Antipoliomylitic Substance in Milk from Human Beings and Certain Cows," ***American Journal of Diseases of Children, 80***, p. 866. (As early as 1950, Dr. Albert Sabin, a discoverer of polio vaccine, reported an antipolio substance in the milk of cows, despite the fact that cows do not get poliomylitis.)

Sabin, Albert B., *et al.*, (1962), "Antipoliomylitic Activity of Human and Bovine Colostrum and Milk," ***Pediatrics, 29***, pp. 105-115. (By 1962, Dr. Sabin had isolated antipolio antibodies in bovine colostrum which were effective against polio in humans.)

Salih, Y., *et al.*, (1987), "Mineral Content of Milk, Colostrum and Serum as Affected by Physiological State and Mineral Supplementation," ***Journal of Dairy Science***, Vol. ***70***, No. ***3***, pp. 608-612. (Colostrum is higher than milk in magnesium, copper, zinc, selenium, iron and phosphorus. Milk is higher in manganese than colostrum.)

Sanchez, L., *et al.*, (1988, "Concentration of Lactoferrin and Transferrin throughout Lactation in Cow's Colostrum and Milk," ***Biological Chemistry Hoppe-Seyler, 369(9)***, pp. 1005-1008. (Highest concentration of both substances was found in the first milking, decreasing sharply through the colostral period, then decreasing more slowly.)

Sandholm, M., *et al,*. (1979), "Colostral Trypsin-Inhibitor Capacity in Different Animal Species," ***Acta Veterinaria Scandinavica***, Vol. ***20***, No. ***4***, pp. 469-476. (Colostrum was found to contain a powerful trypsin-inhibitor which protects colostrum immunoglobulins from digestion.)

Scott, R., Scott, M. and Toms, G.L., (1985), "Cellular Reactivity to Respiratory Syncytial Virus in Human Colostrum and Breast Milk," ***Journal of Medical Virology***, Vol. ***17***, No. ***1***, pp. 83-93. (Role of colostral cellular reactivity in the protection of breast-fed infants from RS virus bronchiolitis is discussed.)

Schweigert, F.J. and Zucker, H. (1988), "Transfer of Beta-Carotene into Colostrum in the Cow," ***International Journal for Vitamin & Nutrition Research***, Vol. ***58***, No. ***2***, pp. 246-247.

Spik, Genevive, *et al.*, "Bacteriostasis of a Milk-Sensitive Strain of E. Coli by Immunoglobulilns and Iron-Binding Proteins in Association," ***Immunology***, Vol. ***35***, No. ***4***, pp. 663-670. (French doctors showed that a combination of IgG and iron-binding protein was bacteriostatic for E. coli.)

Sporn, M.B., *et al.*, (1983), "Polypeptide Transforming Growth Factors Isolated from Bovine Sources and Used for Wound Healing in Vivo," ***Science, 219***, pp. 1329-1331.

(Growth factors in colostrum were found very effective in promoting wound healing.)

Staroscik, Krystyna, *et al.*, (1983), "Immunologically Active Nonapeptide Fragment of a Proline-Rich Polypeptide from Bovine Colostrum: Amino Acid Sequence and Immunoregulatory Properties," ***Molecular Immunology***, Vol. ***20***, No. ***12***, pp. 1277-1282. (Regulates immune system by stimulating underactive system and suppressing overactive system. PRP also appears to act on T-cell precursors to produce helper T-cells and suppressor T-cells. Effect is similar to that of thymus hormones.)

Swarbrick, E.T., (1980), "The Handling of Ingested Antigens," in ***The Immunology of Infant Feeding***, published by Plenum Press, NY, pp. 13-20. (Dr. Swarbrick discovered that during the first 24-36 hours of a newborn's life the bowel wall has a number of large open pores through which big immunoactive molecules from colostrum enter the system.)

Theodore, Christine, *et al.*, (1982), ***Immunologic Aspects of Colostrum and Milk,*** "Development of Antibody Response to Respiratory Syncytial Virus and Bovine Serum Albumin in the Human and Rabbit Mammary Gland," published by Raven Press, New York. (People and animals exposed to Syncytial virus, often responsible for bronchitis and pneumonia, developed IgA and IgG antibodies against this virus in their colostrum.)

Tortora, Gerard; Funke, B. and Cast, C., (1982), "Specific Defenses of the Host: Immunology," in ***Microbiology***, published by Benjamin/Cumming Publishing Co., pp. 403-405. (B-cells of the immune system produce immunoglobulins/antibodies. IgE is associated with allergic reactions.)

Tyrrell, David (1980), "Breast Feeding and Virus Infections," in ***The Immunology of Infant Feeding***, published by Plenum Press, NY, pp. 55-61. (The major benefit of immune factors from colostrum was shown to be their protective activity in the lumen and on the walls of the bowel and bronchials, which means that people of all ages may benefit from colostrum.)

Von Fellenberg, R. and Hoeber, H. (1980), "Multiple Protease Inhibitors in Colostrum and in Bovine Udder Tissue and Their Possible Significance," ***Schweiz. Arch. Tierheilkd.***, Vol. ***122***, No. ***3***, pp. 159-168. (Protease inhibitors in colostrum shut down the digestive enzymes that would normally digest proteins such as the immunoglobulins, allowing them to remain active as they pass into the bowel.)

Wada, N., *et al.*, (1980), "Neutralizing Activity Against Clostridium Difficile Toxins in the Supernatants of Cultured Colostral Cells," ***Infection and Immunity, 29***, pp. 545-550. (Colostrum immune factors neutralize crude toxins from clostridium.)

Weldham, R.H., *et al.*, (1983), "Oral Route as Method for Immunizing Against Mucosal Pathogens," ***Annals of New York Academy of Sciences, 409***, pp. 510-515. (Most infectious diseases enter the body through or remain localized on mucosal surfaces.)

Welsh, J.K., *et al.*, (1976), "Use of Semli Forest Virus to Identify Lipid Mediated Antiviral Activity and Antialphavirus Immunoglobulin A Human Milk," ***Infection and Immunity, 1***, pp. 395-401. (IgA antibodies in colostrum were effective against some alphaviruses.)

Yamamoto, A.; Wada, O. and Suzuki, H., (1988), "Purification and Properties of Biologically-Active Chromium Complex from Bovine Colostrum," ***Journal of Nutrition***, Vol. ***118***, No. ***1***, pp. 39-45. (This colostrum-derived chromium complex is similar to the glucose tolerance factor in yeast and to the chromium-binding substance in mammalian liver.)

If You've Enjoyed Reading This Book . . .

Vibrant Health From Your Kitchen—One of Dr. Jensen's latest and greatest books. In this book, he teaches the basics of health and nutrition. A food guide for family health and well-being. The reader learns how proper foods can overcome certain mineral deficiencies, allergies and build immunity.

Tissue Cleansing Through Bowel Management—Toxic-laden tissues can become a breeding ground for disease. Elimination organs, especially the bowel, must be properly taken care of. This book tells the reader how. Bowel management through a balanced nutritional program with adequate fiber in the diet and regular exercise can often do wonders. A special 7-day cleanse will bring back energy, regenerate tissues and allow good food to let nature do its healing work.

Unfoldment of the Great Within—This new book presents some of the teachings of Dr. V.G. Rocine, together with Dr. Jensen's thoughts and philosophy. In learning ease of mind, we begin to push disease out of our bodies. We should know how to start a new life and new day to become a wiser, healthier and better person.

Chlorella, Jewel of the Far East—Chlorella is a complete food. It is possibly the most thoroughly researched food of our time. One day man will learn to live in harmony with nature. Then we will see a great restoring work being done on this planet, but until that day comes, chlorella is one of the most effective foods to protect us against the toxic effects of pollution.

Herbs: Wonder Healers—Herbalism is at least 5,000 years old, and the effects of many herbs have been carefully documented, especially in China. Health is found in herbs more specifically than in all the other foods we usually purchase. More and more people are using herbs to help reverse and prevent ailments and diseases. Don't take anything for granted about herbs. Get your copy of this wonderful book; read it, and know your herbs.

Foods That Heal—In the first half of this book, Dr. Jensen focuses on the philosophy and ideas of Hippocrates, the brilliant work of Dr. V. G. Rocine, and concludes with a look at his own pioneering work in the field of nutrition. The second half is a nutritional guide to fruits and vegetables.

Juicing Therapy—Health through nature's most natural methods. How nature heals body organs and systems. Wonderful juice combination recipes. Juices for babies and children, soups, herbal green drinks, salad dressings. Special Analytical Food Guide chart.

Garlic Healing Powers—This book contains valuable information on how garlic plays such an important role as a member of the herbal kingdom. It includes garlic research, updates and uses as well as garlic recipes and other ways to enjoy garlic. You can also learn how to treat your family pets with the use of garlic.

Check at your local bookstore for information on Dr. Jensen's books and food products; if they cannot supply them, you may order directly from our office. For a *free* catalog of all his books and supplies, you may write to:

Bernard Jensen International
24360 Old Wagon Road
Escondido, CA 92027